T0110895

FUGITIVE...
FREE THE WAY OUT

JOSH ADAMS

WESTBOW
PRESS®
A DIVISION OF THOMAS NELSON
& ZONDERVAN

WestBow Press books may be ordered through
booksellers or by contacting:

WestBow Press
A Division of Thomas Nelson & Zondervan
1663 Liberty Drive
Bloomington, IN 47403
www.westbowpress.com
844-714-3454

Scripture taken from the New King James Version® Copyright ©
1982 by Thomas Nelson. Used by permission. All rights reserved.

ISBN: 978-1-6642-0881-0 (sc)
ISBN: 978-1-6642-0880-3 (e)

Print information available on the last page.

WestBow Press rev. date: 11/10/2020

Preface

Who am I?

This is my story—my experiences and confession to you—
as a man who wanted to do it right, but ended up in the gutter
anyway. I write this little and simple book to help others in
my situation, just as it was passed on to me. It doesn't matter
if you're in prison or a freeman, a sinner or a saint. This is
about the heart—something we all have and are experts in.

On the outside I tried to seem alright, to fit in, to be respected
as a man…and even feared a little. On the inside, however, I
always felt less-than, a loser, a fake. Like Dr. Jekyll and Mr.
Hyde, I was living a double life. So I tried even harder to play
the role of how I wanted to "be" and feel, of how I wanted
others to see me. As a young man I got big and strong, got
an education, I studied my religion, I served my country, I
got married and had a family. I was checking off all the right
boxes. …And then I crashed.

I suddenly felt unbearably empty, and so I found myself
doing things I never believed I would do. And really liking
them. Confused and conflicted—but also excited—I told
myself I was finally a success, finally fulfilled. High on the
buzz that my new-found life gave me, I eagerly pursued it
and its "fixes" all the more. I felt alive and passionate like

never before. I felt stronger and in control like never before. I was a real big shot, my own way. I was the envy of the other men. I was finally on top!

Meanwhile, I still tried to keep things together on the outside: with my family, friends, work, and community. But it seemed that no one really understood—or *appreciated*—the man I had finally become. And I told myself that it was their fault. I said it was *they* who drove me to do this: to look for something that I needed but that they (my family and friends) were not giving me. I had to be the real man that I felt I finally was. I had a right to this, and I was not about to let anyone take it from me. I felt I was finally breaking free. …And it almost killed me and those closest to me. I couldn't understand it. What the…?!

Nowhere to run, no way to climb out of this pit. Just when I felt I was at the top of my game on the inside, I realized it was also destroying me and my relationships. **Why wasn't my life working?!** Why couldn't I have *both* this newfound "freedom" and the rest of what mattered in my life? I couldn't figure it out. But I also knew I could not get out of this. I couldn't—and really didn't want to—give it up. I just wanted everything *else* to be alright. But I couldn't go back: I was changed for good. There was no way to get my arms around it and put that genie back in the bottle.

It was just like an addiction, quicksand that I could not get out of. No matter what I tried, nothing worked or made sense of my predicament. I became desperate. I sought to move far away. I saw doctors, took meds, joined groups, and prayed. I learned some things, and some of it seemed to work…for a while. But nothing fixed my situation, and I was actually becoming more confused. The further I went along, the more people seemed different, like strangers to me. Why couldn't I just be me...and why couldn't people accept me for what I was? The frustration drove me even harder to get my fixes. But this just exacerbated my depressions, highs, anxiety, and desperation. I was on a wild rollercoaster ride with no end in sight. Why was I losing everything on the outside, when I felt like superman on the inside? Why was my inner soul dying? Why couldn't I get balance? Why couldn't I get it to work? Why was I losing everyone and everything I had loved? Was I dying? Was I going insane?

After struggling for a long time like a thrashing gladiator, I finally became exhausted and admitted that I was defeated. I couldn't see how or why I was still alive. I had no more energy or will to keep fighting. I was through. I stopped looking for any more solutions. I would just play out my losing cards till the bitter end. Just a lost soul, drifting and sinking deeper. Where were the promises? Where was the success? Where was God? And where does a man go from here? The emptiness was unbearable...on all levels.

That was about the time I was yanked out from the gutter... by my neck. Was it friends? Was it some Higher Power like God? Was it fate? All I know is that when all my hope of how I would get better was gone and I stopped trying, I found the answer. Perhaps that's what it took in order for me to become open to such a life-changing answer.

If you can identify with my experiences at all, let me share with you what happened. It's my gift to you and I have to give it away, just like it was a gift to me. You and I are more alike than we can imagine. Then, you, too, can pass it on. No one else can do that like you can.

I have written in short chapters. There is not necessarily a logical progression of one chapter to another. Rather, you may find that some things are repeated from time to time. This is intended to be a genuine, "unofficial," non-professional, and personal sharing of the profound answers I discovered from my inner journey—those that turned my life around, the life that I was convinced was hopeless.

I point out that I am not a certified expert or professional at healing or therapy. I am not a theologian or minister or doctor. And I definitely do not pretend that this is a substitute for seeking the help of such professionals, as well as the help from available programs. I am grateful to all of these and recommend seeking them out when necessary, because they have helped me tremendously to get better, to get sane and sound. What I talk about here is what I have learned on my personal journey, from others and from God. Although I write and make references like a Christian, I am not trying to promote any belief system here—I am merely writing with my own words, from my personal perspective. And I believe anyone can benefit from my experiences. So do not let any religious-sounding or controversial words be an obstacle to you; any biblical cites are just meant to help with extra clarification. What I am talking about here is, for me, beyond the notion of religion or philosophy or creed: It's about the *real* thing. It gets down to the core of being a human. For me, it deals with the very heart of the human soul and mind.

Also, I am writing in the style of one man addressing another, because it helps me express myself more easily.

However, I am writing for everyone—men *and* women—as a brother and fellow traveler. Therefore, do not let any male-sounding references turn you away. That is not my intention. Likewise, if you disagree with any content or feel I have erred in any way (religion, life, view-point, grammar, etc.), forgive me and do not let my shortcomings prevent you from receiving as much benefit as possible.

Will this work, will it help? Yes. It worked for me and many more like me. Because of what I share here, I am no longer a fugitive in my own mind, a loser to myself; no longer confused and frustrated with life. It has led me to a profound joy and peace of mind, even during the hard times: life has become more doable. And it will work for you, too. Afterall, we share the same human nature. Remember, you are not alone.

Your brother,

Josh Adams

Brothers in Christ, Victorious Soldiers Never Alone

We are created for intimate connection. All the time. Our deepest, most basic yearning is to be desired. And when we feel like this is lacking, we do all sorts of absurd things.

How does it feel to know that God is head-over-heals wildly in love with you, to the point that He is giving you His power? If you are reading this, my brother, that means it *is* true for you, and He's been asking me to let you know. It is as real as you are. You were meant to know this.

Now you know it more directly. I had to tell you, because this work is a direct result of my having fallen in love (yes, in love) with God and coming alive all over again through people just like you. We may not know each other, but I know you are reading this. So yeah, it is for *you* that I am writing this, in order to share this impossible but super-real love and power with you too, my brother...in a very healthy mighty way.

Let me let you in on a life-changing secret, one that is a *fact:* We have a greater bond than even soldiers who are fighting in the trenches together. It may be an invisible bond, but it is completely real. Just like gravity, you do not have to see it or understand it to know that it is a real force in your life.

1

God gets you and me through the overwhelming, terrifying, and seemingly hopeless situations in this life by knowing that we are walking together and by just taking the next step with each other. When soldiers fight together in battle, they usually can't see each other because they are marching side-by-side. We draw our strength not from our feelings or the stories in our head, but from simply accepting the reality that we are invincible together. We remain strong and confident and continue to do the next right thing, in spite of how things *seem* to us right now. That's what separates the men from the boys.

Yeah, at times it seems scary and all we want to do is run away and feel better. But courage and manhood are about getting up and moving on, especially in the middle of the fear and pain. You've *already* got what it takes—you are a man, in God's image, and nothing can change that. You already believe in gravity and behave like it is real—you will do the same with this battle, too, step by step and one day at a time. It is with this faith in God's love and power and in our strong brotherhood that we more than win every battle we fight (Romans 8:37). Remember: doing battle is not supposed to feel good, but the rewards and celebration together more than make up for it.

This is a sacred relationship we have with God and each other. No need to talk about it or understand it, just accept it and be grateful. And no matter what, keep getting up and taking the next step. Before you know it, you'll be through it…with your brothers right next to you all the way.

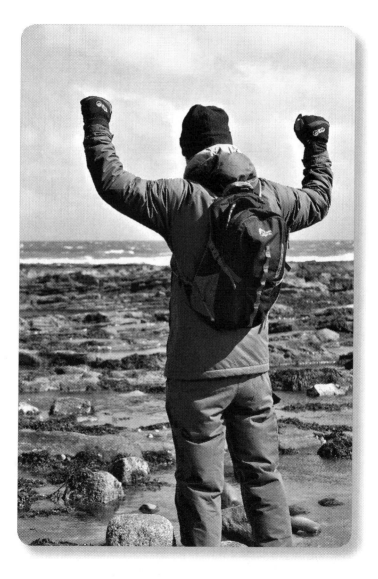

Victorious Personal Commission

Stand and rejoice! You personally (yes, you yourself) have been given a divine and eternal COMMISSION! A trusted charge, awesome privilege, and the most amazing mission from the One Who created the universe…and you. Jesus Christ, the Son of God Himself, paid dearly with his own body and blood in order for you and me to have this in a personal and real way. Therefore, you *are* qualified and worthy of this all-important purpose, this charge, that will make a *huge* difference both in heaven and on earth. He "commissioned" each one of us to be real and true partakers—and therefore active and dynamic agents—in promoting His Kingdom.

God the Father created each one of us separately and with a specific and ***vital*** purpose in mind, which no one other than our own selves—you and I as the individual persons we are—could ever fulfill on earth and in all of human history. We are each created differently as unique persons, living through our own distinct circumstances that shape us to be active agents with personalized, life-changing missions. In this respect, God made us so He could live intimately within us and work through us in a very unique way according to who we (and only *we ourselves*) are. No one else can replace you or me. He created us individually *through* His Son:

As holy John the evangelist says in his gospel: *"All things were made through Him [Jesus, the Word], and without Him nothing was made that was made. In Him was life, and the life was the light of men...[A]s many as received Him, to them* **He gave the right to become children of God***...who were born...of God."* (John 1:3-4, 12-13)

God continues to work for our salvation. And even more, He works *through us* for the good of His Kingdom and for the salvation of those whom we touch in our own way (or rather, whom *He* touches through us). Therefore, He works through each one of us in an individual way and with a specific purpose tailored for us personally—the exact people we are right now. As Saint Paul emphasizes, *"...[A]ll things work together for good to those who love God."* (Romans 8:28) He did not pay the ultimate and inconceivable price for us to be mere bystanders in this life trying to figure out our way, our mission, on our own. Actually, he did this to restore us to His Kingdom, His world and reality. He had each one of us personally on His mind and with His heart yearning indescribably for each one of us. ...To live dynamically (energetically and with passion) through us. Jesus himself pointed out that, *"indeed, the kingdom of God is within you."* (Luke 17:21)

This shows very clearly that God has truly commissioned each of us personally to work for the good and advancement of His Kingdom, which also means for our own good. This "commission" is as *real* as real can be! And it is an inconceivable privilege. We are much more than worldly commissioned officers in a prestigious service for a while, for a mere career, where we hope to make a difference and be relevant in some way. Rather, we are *co-workers* with Jesus

Christ himself and co-heirs with him of the eternal Kingdom of God. (Romans 8:16-17) He is bringing His Kingdom through each and every one of us! That is an honor beyond our imagination. And it is eternal...and most real!

So, how do we actually participate in God's will and carry out this incredible commission? We do this by simply doing the next right thing that is in front of us to do. We leave the outcomes to God—He has the playbook. We also ask Him to teach us humility (that is, a right attitude based on truth) and to give us the strength to do the next right thing. God will take it from there and grow us with further understanding. That is why when we pray, we should put our requests within the context of the good for God's Kingdom as well as for our salvation, which is the whole of His desire. In other words, we tell God, "*Your* will, not mine, be done." This is how it was revealed to a well-known nun, who was a spirituality-television pioneer commissioned by God to spread this good news, when she had asked the Lord why it seemed that He did not grant some of her prayers: She heard God explain to her that some of her specific requests would not be good for her, nor for His Kingdom (that is, for the rest of us).

All of this means that we no longer need to struggle to find our place and make something meaningful of ourselves, *all on our own.* We no longer have to wonder if we are good enough, or if we can make the grade. We no longer need to fight obsessively to prove ourselves and frantically strive for a "sense" of fulfillment. We now have the answer to our eternal and most burning question, the fulfillment of our deepest daily desire and yearning, and the goal of our most core drive: We are Kingdom Men! We are *alive* for the Kingdom of God, vibrant and uniquely vital members.

We truly are sons of God, in our flesh and in our soul, through whom He advances His Kingdom. Our status has been guaranteed by the blood of Jesus and can never be undone. As Saint Paul points out, Jesus has already died for us and risen, once and for all, and he cannot die again. (Romans 6:9-10, 8:38-39) That means it cannot be changed or undone—it's permanent for you and me. Therefore, our mission is guaranteed for success, and nothing can prevent it as long as we are willing to keep taking our steps with God.

Let us, then, man-up and act the part, as individuals and to each other. What does this look like? In everything, we invite God to use us today, right now—in everything we do—for our salvation and for the good of His Kingdom. We can say a simple prayer like, "Lord, be with me!" or "Lord, help me remember that you are with me right now." And we talk plainly to Him throughout the day—He is more than eager to hear us in our own words. We continue to do this throughout the day and night as we go through our routine, as well as in every unexpected situation.

We have found our ultimate mission and reason to live: We are God's directly-commissioned servants and partners in everything we do this day, and we matter beyond our understanding. "For we are God's fellow workers." (1 Corinthians 3:9)

Congratulations, you and I are finally free! WE ARE FINALLY FREE OF OUR OWN DEVICES. For Good. Yes, Lord, come!

P.S. Something more you should know…

With this new awareness and attitude—even if just making a beginning—we are now open and accepting of GRACE. Grace means no longer accusing or suspecting ourselves—nor having fears about ourselves—that we may somehow be recognized as being *wrong* or *not enough* in some way. That used to make us "feel" naked, shameful, and afraid; wanting to hide, flee, avoid, and to take matters into our hands to cover up and medicate. Now, we accept ourselves ALWAYS as God sees us: freed and reconciled of any wrongness by His Grace, as confirmed through the permanent and irretractable gift of His Son Jesus Christ. We now step forward and march on as true men of God, finally and forever free!

Human Nature: Born To Be Divine

Biologically, we are endowed with a mind that is aware of something greater than ourselves, and a desire to reach higher. To reach for the stars. Human psychology has studied this a lot.

According to religion, we are uniquely endowed with the Spirit of our Creator. Our own mind constantly proves to us that we were never made to be by ourselves, just in ourselves—we could never stand that. Since every human has a psyche, a "soul," it means we have a spirit (the "image" of our Creator). And since God *is* love (the purest and perfect expression of spirit), it logically follows that we were made "to be loved"—to share intimately in the spirit of God. This is the "God-sized" hole that we yearn to be filled at our deepest level, to make us feel perfectly whole like we were created to be.

It is therefore natural for us to seek and yearn in our core for something greater, to make something "more" of ourselves. We have the ability to make comparisons and to judge what we think is the value of ourselves…and we react to it. This is part of our innate "free will."

But when we honestly look at ourselves, by ourselves, we human beings have to admit that, on our own, we are rather marginal; that as individuals in ourselves, we are actually unremarkable, not extraordinary.

This conclusion, however, goes against our most basic, natural, and in-born wiring; it runs counter to our instinctual sense of self-awareness, of what we *should* be. We are deeply, perhaps even unconsciously, aware of greater potential for ourselves—we all instinctively know we must contend for something more. And we cannot live with just being who and what we believe we are at the present.

We compare ourselves with others and other standards, either real or perceived...and we always fall short. We believe the lie and the story that we are not enough, not "right." Furthermore, our God-created mind is also conscious of time, and we often draw conclusions based on this: We are afraid, scared to the core, about our future...and also afraid to admit it. We believe we are not enough and cannot *definitely* secure and guarantee our own future to become "right," to be "successful." We feel an overwhelming, imperious, and all-pervasive "need" to take matters into our hands. We end up living in an illusion about ourselves and about the meaning of our lives based on these stories we tell ourselves. We have no other option but to believe that this self-induced "fantasy" is actually our reality. Why? Because our mind naturally resorts to this since we lack an "objective" sense of reality (our mind can only draw its own "subjective" conclusions). We therefore lack the genuine and *undeniable* sense of self-worth that is both inherent to us and inalienable from us—that is, nothing can change it or take it away from us because that is how we were created: Being loved as perfect is our birthright. (Romans 8:16) This is also the only way that God—as perfect Spirit and Creator—relates to us: in perfect and unconditional love. And since God is unchangeable, nothing can change that about Him...or *us*. Therefore, the idea in our minds that we are not right enough is merely a perversion (a misleading twist) from the truth. But it is a very powerful one when we believe it, one that ultimately brings ruinous consequences in our lives because our thoughts and actions are based on a very defective view. Perhaps this un-truth is why the name of evil, the devil, means one who distorts and twists the truth.

To make matters worse, our culture and upbringing strongly reinforce the notion that we must make something "more" of ourselves: that we are masters of our own destiny; that we are responsible for our own success; that, otherwise, we are failures and abnormal, "less-than."

We therefore succumb to the calls and the clever marketing to "improve" ourselves. We often try to attain this through our own achievements. We are motivated to succeed in this respect, and it often becomes an obsession and overwhelming motivator. We suffer in deep yearning to "connect" with something, or someone, to make us feel whole and right. We feel we cannot live without it.

At the end of the day, however, we are aware that we are still ourselves, that nothing has changed about who we are essentially, on the inside. Knowing no other way out, this drives us to desperation and to commit irrational acts. We run, we medicate, we hurt others. These, in turn, only deepen our sense of worthlessness and failure.

Then…we finally hit bottom and become open and willing to try anything that may help. We are led to the conclusion that we cannot make our own selves better or more complete. We are willing to move out of the way, and to invite God in.

This change of mindset, this "metanoia," allows us to see ourselves through God's eyes, objectively and truthfully. This is the basic word Jesus preached when he went around the towns pleading with the people, "Repent [metanoia], for the kingdom of heaven is at hand." (Matthew 4:17) He is asking us to change our mindset and let God's reality ("kingdom") replace our lying stories so we can finally be free and complete. As psychologists know, when we change the stories that we tell ourselves about ourselves, then we change our reality. More than anything, God understands our personal situation and accepts us exactly as we are; He knows we can do no more on our own. So He comes to us individually and is encouraging us to let go and accept the truth, the good news, the "gospel" that we can now let God's reality come inside us and free us. This change of mindset, this "letting-go," makes it possible. This is where we see the truth that with Him we are perfect as we are and perfectly loved, because we are made in His divine image, endowed with His Spirit. We can accept the truth that we are His entire universe, and that He alone loves us unconditionally and yearns for us personally beyond everything else.

We realize that as His creation, and in His holy image, and endowed with His very own spirit, we are already perfect and complete. Nothing can ever change this reality. Only the lie that we are not enough has deceived us to believe that we are unwanted, unloved, and a failure. It is the most fundamental lie that goes against the most basic truth of our existence, of our very nature. And we cannot live with that. At least not peacefully. Only the truth of God's love, which was proven through the sacrifice of His only Son for us personally, reveals the truth most powerfully. And we feel complete only when we are connected to this truth, which in actuality connects us to Him.

This faith and believing, therefore, sets us free and connects us with the Truth of our completeness and wholeness. Only through believing in His unconditional love and perfect esteem for us through His Son are we truly "made" free and complete. Freedom, then, is a matter of personal faith, of mindset (metanoia). This is how we have been created, and we are truly "free" and alive to the fullest of our natural potential by accepting God's Truth, turning away from the lie that we are not enough: Accepting God's spirit and love and image and His being within our very essence. We were created naturally for intimate co-existence with our creator God (theosis). All we have to do to "actuate" it, to be free and complete once and for all, is to believe it—or at least be *willing* to believe it and asking for God's help. God will then do the rest; He always does. Wise people before us have passed on this liberating principle of daily living: We merely take the next step and do the next right thing; however it turns out is how it is supposed to be.

This total surrender to God's truth, to the truth of our very essence, means that we no longer are in a position to judge ourselves. We surrender ourselves to God; we surrender our judgment and self-judgment to His unconditional love. It is only right that we do so—He paid a very dear price for it. He gave up everything for each of us to accept it and be free; we owe Him at least the same. Such sacrifice and surrender is the expression of Truth and Love. It is being true to our human nature.

In our lives and human experience, this takes constant, daily effort and struggle. As essentially "relational" beings, we need to foster this truth through fellowship and personal relationship with God and our fellow man. We start by simple honest prayer: talking to God with complete and humble honesty, and showing simple kindness to others. Like a loving and caring personal coach and father, He will do the rest. We just take the next small step and leave the big picture to Him who is all-powerful and all-faithful to us. So relax, let go, and be *free!* What do you have to lose?

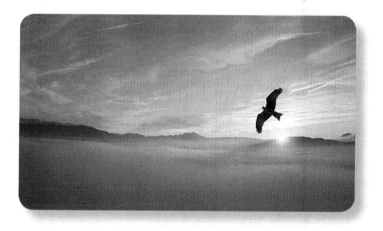

Why Does My Program Fail?

Why do most of my attempts to break free from unhealthy habits, or to change my life in some way, ultimately fail? I often find that it is because I still hold on to my *own* concept of what successful living is, of what "being healed" and "being right enough" is supposed to look like for me; I keep my own picture of it in my mind, instead of keeping an open mind about it. Whether or not I am healed or overcome all my harmful habits is not the final point of my struggle or program. What *I* want and what *I* think this change should look like, and when *I* think it should happen, is not always feasible, or even the most beneficial for me. Nor is it necessarily God's will for me and what is truly best for me in the end. Moreover, healing is often more about the personal growth—and the miracles—that happen along the way. (Saints Paul and James say it very well in Romans 5:3, and James 1:2-4) And I'm usually clueless at the start about what the journey will actually do for me and for those around me—about the life-changing gifts it always brings, and in ways I could not have imagined.

If one day I were to believe that I have been automatically healed or perfected exactly the way that I think it should look like (that is, on my terms and along my way of thinking), it would mean that I no longer would need to have a faith that is a "total" dependence on God's mercy for my redemption (my ultimate and *true* healing). If I believe that I fully know the paradigm—the model—for what "healed" means, then I am not trusting God completely; instead, I am proceeding according to my own and imperfect judgments, both of God and of myself. I am selling short God and his ways, as well as the potential of my own life. What a waste that would be—I deserve much better than that!

It is easy for the temptation to come and convince me with the lie that "it" (my program, my new way) does not work, and that I am ultimately a failure. In my frustration, then, I am misled to believe that it is no use for me to try any longer. I let myself become like an athlete who has amazing potential but gives up because of his failures...the same failures that could (and would) lead to his best development, if only he would keep going. All of the best athletes, saints, and the other truly "successful" people have had many missed goals (even embarrassing ones) and set-backs, all the time. But they understood that this was actually part of the process of becoming a great person, and they manned-up and kept getting up and putting one foot in front of the other in order to let the benefit come. Without occasional more weight or resistance, one cannot build muscle or endurance; without more practice, one cannot grow their skills and get even better at what they do. So it is with *all* of us. Like those examples for us, our "heroes," it is not about merely achieving a specific goal that we may have in mind; rather, it is more about the great things we accomplish and the inspiration we give as we stay in the game. And our success—whatever that may look like—is guaranteed. (Romans 5:3-4, 8:37; Hebrews 12:1-11) Often, though, we are "heroes" without realizing it at the moment.

The point for me, then, is not to give up and not to stay down. But rather, to keep getting up and continuing on the road, trusting only in God's unconditional love for me. If I believe that having a fall means I am a failure, then that self-defeating attitude based on my self-definition of "success and healing" will eventually trip me up in despair and loss of faith. It will actually harm me, because it will drive me to more desperation and seeking to medicate in any way possible. It will not allow me to grow as I need to, to accept God's true healing and redemption for me and let Him actually turn that negative into a positive for me. I have to let it become a "positive" opportunity for me, one that grows me and makes me stronger. God can and *will* do this for me if I let Him, if I just keep going and doing the next right thing (Romans 8:28.) Just like the athletes who learn from their falls and get up and continue their practice.

The key for me, therefore, is to always get up and keep going; never despair and lose faith...and always believe in (accept as *real*) God's unconditional love and redemption, no matter how it feels to me or what I think about it at the time. My own way of thinking, even with the best intentions, is often neither the best nor what God desires for me. (I can just look at how well my own way has worked for me so far.) I must rely only and ultimately on Him and His grace. What I think is *im*-possible, is indeed possible for God. (Mark 9:23, 10:27) That's just the way He works: bringing something good out of something bad, always...if I get out of the way and let Him. This is what's behind *true* obedience. I used to dislike that word ("obedience"), thinking that it meant letting someone else impose their own will over mine and make me a weak slave that submits to their way. That's because I did not grow up learning the correct meaning of obedience: trusting one who knows better than I do and wants the best for me. Just like a small child trusts and obeys—and depends upon—his caring parents, guardians, and teachers who he knows would never harm him and are always there to help him grow the best way possible because they love him and know more than he does; and who also protect him and see him through all the difficulties because they are able to do so. Obedience in this sense is about *freedom* from problems. Additionally, I'm willing to trust others all the time without even thinking about it: doctors, mechanics, pilots, bus drivers, etc. Why, then, would I not trust the Almighty Who has shown me that He loves me more than His own child? In a similar way, those preconceived notions and plans and programs that I have—if these ideas *in themselves* become the ultimate measure of my healing—only end up taking the place of my ultimate healer: God! I therefore keep an open mind with God (not my own ideas) as the *driver* of my program and my entire life. I bring *Him* into all my life programs. He has already proven over and over that He will never fail or abandon me, and that He has already guaranteed my success.

Faulty Reflections

As humans with a soul or psyche which is not made up of matter and is indefinable, we naturally yearn at our core to reach and connect with something "more," something "other," something "higher." As we have been trained in the world, we try to do this using our own understanding, ideas, and assumptions. But we are not omnipotent—the created cannot comprehend the creator on its own. The desire to do so may be there, but it is beyond our own reach and abilities.

Moreover, we have limited abilities that cannot understand all of reality. As many wise people have concluded, we are essentially spiritual beings (that is, we have a psyche, a soul not of this world) who are living a worldly human experience. We can only understand—and therefore accept or believe—what our brain (our "mind") can fathom as reality. Our concept of reality, therefore, is based on what our brain can generate about it. Since all things in this "subjective reality" of ours are conceived (fashioned, "created") out of our own minds, we naturally make ourselves—without even realizing it—the God of that "reality." This means that unwittingly, we have pushed the real, the spiritual and true, God out.

In our attempt to see things rightly and fit in, we naturally project our own ways and thinking onto our concept of

God. This has been done naturally throughout the entire human history. But our concept of right and wrong and righteousness is inadequate, based primarily on our own experiences. We naturally assume that God is like we are, and that he judges like we do and therefore condemns us. But nothing could be further from the truth! That doesn't even make sense, since God is pure love beyond our understanding. And love does not condemn. (John 3:17) As a simple and holy spiritual father of our time has said, from his own personal experience with God:

> This is the way we should see Christ—he is our friend, our brother. He is whatever is good and beautiful. He is everything. Yet he is still a friend and he shouts it out, "You're my friends to me, don't you understand that? We're brothers. I'm not threatening you. I don't hold hell in my hands. I love you. I want you to enjoy life together with me!" That is the reality of it, of who we (you and I personally) are to God.

Unfortunately, however, when we see our faults, we cannot believe that we are worthy of God's love, nor that we are acceptable and enough in our present condition. We ultimately conclude—wrongly— that God does not love us and that He rejects us. Our experiences with people and the world where we have grown up and live also seem to reinforce this. But this feeling and "belief" runs contrary to our core nature and the way we were created: ***to be one with God***. Desperately using our human reasoning, we try to fix this by attempting to make something "more" of ourselves—to acquire more personal "creds." Nevertheless, what we think we really are continues to be unacceptable to us, and we become more desperate and seek to medicate and run into another reality—to blur out and numb our faulty self-story—but we always end up with ourselves again. As human beings, this translates into greater emotional and physical distress, and ultimately more desperate actions.

In order to make the leap out of this faulty thinking that is destroying our lives, it is necessary to use more than just our own reasoning (the imperfect cannot make itself perfect). This requires faith—we naturally were made to see through *faith*. As previously pointed out, our soul (our core) is not material, and therefore we cannot use earthly means to view its reality. Otherwise, we are blinded from our core truth that we are actually okay and right and perfect in God's eyes. All leaps into a new reality require the creativity of faith that allows us to see and trust in another reality (the actual truth about ourselves), even though we do not fully understand it. But we can still accept it. For example, how do we define love? We know it is very real, but we cannot fully comprehend or define it with our minds. Nevertheless, we *accept* it and live on... And even depend on it. Love is a personal and absolutely real experience. It is of the soul and therefore profound, beyond human reasoning and understanding. Like little children who simply trust their parents or their loving guardians, we can have no peace or serenity—neither emotionally, nor spiritually, nor physically—without FAITH. Faith allows us to see with the mind of our soul.

Jesus Christ, the son of God, came to open our eyes and feed us through faith. He came to show and personally demonstrate once and for all God's unconditional love for each and every one of us, precisely because it is beyond our own concept and thinking. And he did so in very human terms and experiences. So this is not merely something that is abstract teachings or philosophical knowledge to be acquired. Rather, love is about personal relationship and experience. Jesus is real, historically proven, and therefore he is *undeniable proof* of God's love for us and the truth about ourselves. Through him and his sacrifice for us, we have real and foolproof factual evidence that we are undeniably accepted, loved, and right—absolutely guaranteed. By coming into our own human experience on this earth, Jesus the Christ of God has given us a way to believe it and accept this reality about ourselves fully in our own lives, every moment and forever. In other words, God loves us so much that He even sent to us—to our own existence, into our world—His own (and only) child to prove it to us *in person*, so that we would accept it as God-honest truth and never again have any reason to doubt it! (John 3:16) That is, we have historical physical proof of this. We are perfected in symbiosis (life-partnership, union) with Him. And this truth becomes our own reality through faith: that is, by simply accepting it... Just like we accept love, gravity, and the other realities we cannot explain. It is most simple and most basic, not something that can be acquired by any amount of personal achievements or accumulated knowledge. That's why babies don't have to be "taught" to love.

The undeniable existence of our soul—our core—cannot be explained by anything in this world, and, therefore, it could not have come *from* this world. We have been told by countless witnesses throughout human history, who were so absolutely sure about its validity that they readily gave up their worldly lives for this revealed truth: that Christ is the

Logos (Word) of God through whom we were created and upon whom our nature depends. That is, we exist through him. Since God's "Word" and reasoning are beyond that of this world, it alone can explain the existence of our "inexplainable" soul. (John 1:3) Because our soul is *spiritual* and not of this world, its life and energy are created from and dependent upon its source. That is why Christ is called the "Tree of Life." Without him, our own tree of knowledge (our mind and our sense of reality) is inadequate and ultimately leads to death, the natural result of all earthly life: we return to the ground. Jesus, the incarnate (in-the-flesh) Logos of God, is our life! And that Life is beyond anything of this world and therefore cannot die or change. When we accept this and invite him in—through faith—we see the Truth about ourselves and are re-ignited with life in union with our Creator. We don't worry about how this is made possible or what this process must look like—we already know and accept that it is beyond our understanding, that it is about the living experience of our soul. God makes it possible. We just trust and take the next step, moment by moment and day by day. We live with satisfaction and contentment (about ourselves and our "perfect-ness"), with peace and joy, in every single moment: We no longer have to anxiously await and worry and struggle to be deemed "right." That's precisely what faith is about, and why we were meant to live by faith. (Romans 1:17; Galatians 3:11)

Where Does My Religion Fit In?

How do I *live* what I truly believe – my religion and spirituality? Is it like exercise or work that I do only at certain times, like when I pray or go to church? How do I integrate it into my entire life and being... into everything I think, say, and do? In other words, how do I acquire it as a natural mindset, to be my best? Do I have to become a monk, or practice an extremely strict lifestyle? No, that has never worked for me: I lack the faith, perseverance, strength, and motivation to keep up a "pious" attitude and behavior for long. Life in this opposite and corrupted world is full of temptations and conditions—whether within myself or perceived in others—that continuously incite me away from being my best for any respectable length of time. As others have said, it is as if we are constantly breathing poisonous air: No matter how long I try to hold my breath or put on a clean-oxygen mask, I always have to return to the same environment. So, without moving to a monastery or living in some bubble, how can I survive in this state? Should I join a 12-Step or religious group or get a spiritual director? Those are not bad ideas, if you can do it.

Besides the other tools out there that involve reflection, religion, fellowship, and healing growth, I would like to suggest a question: Are you personally living the religion *of* Jesus Christ, or the religion *about* Jesus Christ? Do you have a personal, intimate relationship with Christ Himself, or only with His institutions and principles? The latter are not bad at all, and, in fact, are helpful for sane living and growth. But they will always leave you *thirsty for more*.

Because we are made with this God-sized hole and meant to live united in harmony with God, we will never feel rested and satisfied until our hearts rest in Him (as St. Augustine concluded). Trying to "act it" into reality may be a start, but it's hard to keep it up. The other way is to let go and invite God to come and rest in us. We admit prayerfully and sincerely to God that we cannot do it by ourselves, and we ask Him to come and do this for us and through us. We ask for this continuously, especially after our failures and falls. This is not an end in itself; rather, it is a way of life. <u>Success, therefore, is not a matter of never failing, but of never giving up in spite of our perceived failures</u> (it's about the journey, not the destination).

Jesus did not simply follow a religious regimen or prescribed rules. He unceasingly availed Himself to God the Father to use Him and work through Him. He became a living religion Himself. His religion was not a set of beliefs and actions; rather it is a living person and relationship – God the Father living fully in Him and touching others. When we take the attitude that we are not going to measure our spirituality and "right-ness" by how many items we can check off a list, but instead through our active expression of love to God and toward others, then we are on the road to imitating Christ. Like Jesus, we become not rote imitators of a religion, but living and effectual expressions of our loving Creator and source of Life. ...Wrapped up in one person. God makes that possible, and it is His happy will to do this for us (Luke 12:32).

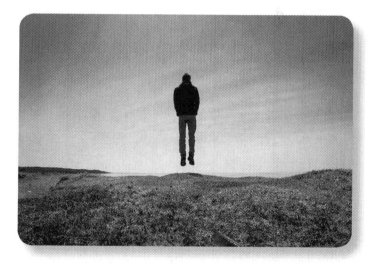

Overcoming the Temptations of Feelings

As humans, we all have feelings. All the time. And we all too often tell ourselves stories based on those feelings—stories that we believe and that shape our reality. We do this automatically, without giving it much thought. When feelings of weakness or lowness or failure strike us, for whatever reason—perceived or real—we often tell ourselves a false story about ourselves and we believe a lie. For example, if I'm feeling down, I may tell myself that I am a "failure." That's because that "feeling" is connected to an intense negative and hurtful experience from our early youth, where we falsely believed there was something *wrong* with us. So for a long time, we have always associated that feeling with a false but painful conclusion about ourselves, about what we are. Now, after many years of practice, we automatically link a mere feeling to a profound and wounding story, one that is not even true. And we become even more convinced of the lie that there is something wrong with us: that we are defective, that we are a failure and "less-than."

The truth, however, is that this is just a human feeling, like a wave or the wind. Something has simply triggered our human chemistry and memory. The sensation is real, but the truth of who we are—good, strong, worthy men of

God—has not changed in spite of how we feel. Just like a rainy day cannot diminish the value of a hero.

The simple way to break this pattern of debilitating lies is to recognize and acknowledge the feeling, but then separate it from any such story we tend to tell ourselves about ourselves. In its place, we invite God in and ask Him for the grace and strength to remain in His company—to see ourselves *in truth*, as He sees us. We do this even when the feeling seems strong and overwhelming. We do not give in to the false story; that would be absurd and wrongly wound us and others. Instead, we simply accept God's spirit, the Paraklete ("Comforter"), the life-giving Spirit of unchangeable Truth...whether we *feel* it or not. The more we practice this, the more automatic it will become.

Even if we slip to medicate the feeling, we are still winners by surrendering any story afterward to God and inviting Him in, so that we remember His holy and real presence with us and unconditional love. The only thing that can convince us otherwise is a total and absurd lie, inconsistent with who we really are by our very nature and birthright: God's beloved. That's why it is so important to recognize the lie and replace it with God's truth, especially after we have done something we think is wrong. Afterall, wrong actions do not make a wrong person. The Holy Spirit is ready to do this for us, anywhere and anytime, and in spite of how impossible it seems. Faith rescues us and can never fail us. Glory to Jesus our Christ, who has already paid every requirement for us and has given us free access to the Holy Spirit, the Truth.

Accepting Adversity
The Deception of FEELING
"Smug, Comfortable"

I have always sought to feel comfortable, to feel like everything is "all right." I erroneously believed the story that life and things are right if they "feel" right. I wasted much of my life, and my ambitions, living by this lie of an axiom: that if it *feels* good, it must *be* good; and that it must *feel* good to *be* good. Now I finally see that the feeling of being comfortable and "smug" is: 1) not about reality, but merely a feeling or perception; and 2) a liability for me that keeps me from maturing and growing stronger emotionally and spiritually.

The reality is that God has my life, and all I need to do is trust in Him. How "it" feels is not the measure of life or my worth. On the contrary, depending upon and striving for a sense of smugness (the feeling that all is under control and just the way I think it should be) sets me up for disillusion and frustration. That's because an attitude of looking to *feel* comfortable is ego-based and ego-driven: it makes me believe erroneously—and even unconsciously—that I can manage my life, and not depend on God. It subtly draws me away from faith and leaves me unprepared to peacefully and rationally handle any coming adversity and difficulty, which is sometimes just around the corner… That's called life: adversity and pain are going to happen; how I respond to them and let them affect me is to a large extent up to me.

The point is not to simply seek to feel comfortable and good; such feelings are often dependent upon and controlled by external events, as well as my internal (psycho-chemical) reaction to what I *think* those events and circumstances mean. Why would I leave my psychological state of balance in the hands of chance and simple emotions like that? That doesn't make sense, and it is not the way I was made to live. As a spiritual being with a human mind, I was meant to keep my focus, my dependence, on the immoveable rock that is God Himself—the same God Who is all-powerful, all-loving and compassionate, and always wants the very best for me; the same One who is in control and will lead me out of "the valley of the shadow of death," even when it feels too difficult and scary for me. All I have to do is tell Him that I leave it up to Him and love Him and ask for His help and strength to just do the next right thing. This may sound like a child's fairytale, but it is nevertheless true. Because God doesn't require complicated things from us: He wants us to trust like innocent children, as Jesus has stressed (Matthew 18:2-4). This allows me to live with an unshakeable inner peace and joy…under any circumstances, even when there is also pain, fear, and sadness. It takes a little practice at first, but the more I practice it, the more it becomes a natural part of my human experience and response to adversity. (Matthew 14:22-33)

So, seeking to feel good is not the way. Rather, I can better depend on God and handle life in a positive and constructive way that actually gives me peace and builds me up if I am willing to accept that it is ok *not* to feel (chemically) comfortable or smug all the time; those feelings quickly vanish, but the peace and internal joy that comes from trusting God is permanent and can see me through all adversity. The more I practice this, the more peaceful I will be...because I will no longer be dependent upon (a slave to) my own feelings, which come and go like the wind, but rather on God's lasting and freeing reality. And I can only do this by FAITH. The more I live by faith—not basing my sense of reality (my sense of whether things are going right or wrong) on FEELINGS—the more I will live free in peace. ACCEPTING adversity when it comes (not running to feel comfortable) and giving it in trust over to God actually grows me spiritually and emotionally, and it makes me stronger to face other challenges in a positive way. That, in turn, will leave me feeling "spiritually good" (truly good on the inside) and confident to handle—together with God—anything that life throws my way. In short, God becomes *everything* for us.

Note: This is not meant to downplay the pain and difficulties that people suffer in their lives, and in the lives of their loved ones. Rather, this is meant as encouragement for one to stay positive, to the extent they are able to do so, during those hard times—to not let the experiences take them down, but instead to receive greater strength to keep on going and living in a peace that will also help others. Sometimes this also means seeking professional help if it is indicated, as well as relying even more on fellowship with friends and loved ones, and practicing our own private spiritual meditation and prayer.

Down... But Not Out

A deep confession to my brothers: I don't understand my difficult moments or feelings, but I find myself in them all too often. And sometimes it seems to be impossible for me to go on. All I want to do is *run*. But somehow, even when I think it's hopeless, God gets me through it—often through the people around me who may not even know what's going on with me. I appreciate your letting me share the following with you—the story of my life. But I'm sure you can relate to it too: The weight of my sinful condition, my sense of desperation and lack of hope and faith, and my overwhelming sense of being a loser is often too much for me to bear. At times it seems that my own mind and body, and the people around me—and even God and His very words—are against me. I feel that I can only resign myself to the fact that I am in a physical and mental decline for good.

I remember and painfully relate to Saint Paul's own words that I continue to do the things that I hate, most wretched man that I am; who will save me? (Romans 7:14-25)

Yeah, but with your help, my brothers, I have learned ***not to let these feelings and stories dictate my reality.*** I may feel knocked down and decimated, but I cannot believe that I am out. I have to just keep putting one foot in front of the other. Even if the healing that *I* want never comes, I must never forget that our Lord Jesus Christ has already won the victory for me, and for you my brothers. I am, therefore, no longer a slave to my sinful physical condition, in spite of what I continue to do. And I can just admit my shortcomings and praise and thank God, and then simply try to do the next right thing. No more judgments. No more trying to fix things. No more fear about my sanity. …All of that has been rendered moot, a non-issue. Unfortunately, few earthlings actually understand and believe this—so I'm so grateful for you guys. And, yes, in some way, I love you. Because living this way requires more strength and faith than is in me.

Thanks for listening. That's _life_, that's the struggle, that's the race—and it's already been won for me (and for *you*)! It's up to me to accept it, to stand up like a man, have faith, and take the next step. That makes me stronger, more confident, and more resilient and useful as I keep going. I am a winner!

Why We Suffer

A friend once explained to me why we experience suffering: It is because God loves us so much. He wants us to be so close to Him. He Himself personally chose each of us out from this world. We are not of this world; therefore, we sometimes feel like we suffer.

But God tells us to take heart! He keeps us close to Himself and gives us His peace, which neither the world nor anything in it or outside it has the power to take away from us. He let us know beforehand that in this world we will have pain, but that He has overcome the world for us. (John 16:33)

He paid an unthinkable price for His love for each of us and will always be with us. So, whether we feel like we live or die, we are the Lord's—nothing has changed (Romans 14:8). To Him be glory and thanksgiving, forever. Amen.

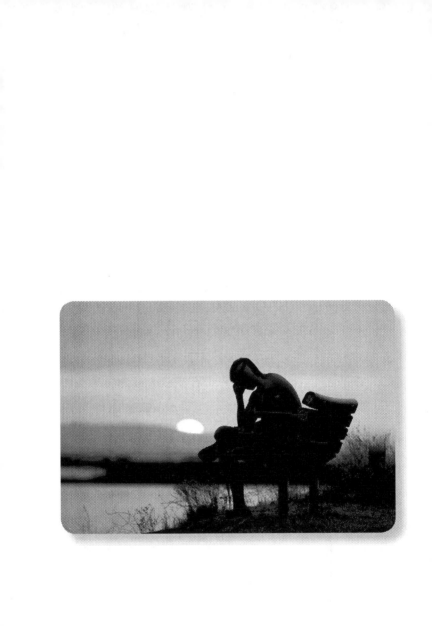

Peace, Not Dis-Comfort

Dis-comfort: the absence of faith; trying to cope by ourselves with something that is bigger than us; trying to comprehend the infinite, by using our limited and imperfect minds; imagining our "reality" and trying to live by our own expectations; depending on our own reasoning, and believing false stories and lies; false self-image; always trying to get there but never satisfied; insecurity and need to control; need to make *ourselves* God, in control of our destinies and the life around us—because we are falsely convinced that we are separated from God, not enough, rejected, not loved; fear, desperation and insanity.

God is above all. He is above every being, every law, every possibility and every conceived "reality." He is pure LOVE, and nothing can disturb Him, because He is not dependent on anything. And the saving miracle that is **already true** for each of us is that *absolutely nothing* can change His personal and un-conditional love for us, ourselves as we are. and his fervent desire and absolute ability to give the best for us. (Romans 8:35-39) Therefore…

LOVE is the absence of disturbance: love is tranquility and peace; trust and sense of security; it is acceptance—of the way things and people are—and surrender: not trying to fight people and life into the way we want them to be, when we want them to be; it is humility (accepting the truth). Accepting we are perfect and enough in Jesus Christ. ...That we are already "there." It takes the constant practice of faith in the unseen, no matter how often we feel scared and down. Courage can only be demonstrated when we feel fear; the same is true for faith. But walking forward in spite of the fear builds a stronger faith and courage, and the result is that we grow in this confidence and can let go of our disturbances. Then, we naturally feel alright, love and loved. Love is PEACE. And God makes that absolutely possible for each of us.

The Hallmark of Manhood

It is not how well we behave when we feel *good* that counts—
it takes no strength or moral fiber to act good when we *feel*
good. The measure of our greatness and character, rather,
is best revealed in how we respond during moments of
suffering, pain, and adversity. In how well we treat others—
and God—and continue to do the right thing, especially
in spite of how we feel. Such spirit and attitude embody
humility, integrity, obedience, courage, and selfless love.
It is the epitome, the standard, of maturity and Manhood.

We are privileged beyond our understanding to have our
Lord Jesus as our prototype, our model. Through his
suffering we've gained freedom, release, boundless joy, and
eternal salvation. Through his voluntary suffering, we've
gained access to perfect maturity, perfect love, and God-
likeness as His real children. (Romans 5:8-9, 8:16) When
we imitate Jesus, we mature and grow *into* him. Moreover,
we miraculously reflect our loving God INTIMATELY to
others: They see and experience God with us.

To do this, we must accept—and even embrace head-on—
suffering as perfectly normal, not something to be avoided
at all cost. Instead of running from it, let's try to surrender
to it and make the best out of it by doing the next right thing.
That's all. Not living in the past with it or thinking about

what it could mean in the future, but just keeping our eyes on the present moment—where God is—and with trembling courage take the next right step. That's what a man with integrity and true strength does. By putting it in God's hands this way and living in *His* moment (*His* reality) where nothing is impossible, we will surely find that the issue is no longer a monster of a problem that overwhelms us, and we can see it in its true light: as something that is definitely doable and will even result ultimately in our good…if we do it together with God. That's just how it works with God. Look at what happened to Jesus' disciple Peter when he was struggling with his brothers in the boat being beaten by the storm: As soon as he put his eyes, his focus, on Jesus in the midst of the scary waves and wind, his problem diminished. And where was Jesus located when Peter looked to him? He was actually walking calmly and with no problem on that stormy water, and he was urging Peter to take courage and to just keep his eyes on him—not to consider only the storm around him and get distracted and overwhelmed with it, but to walk *with* him. When Peter was *willing* to do so—to trust him and take the next step—he saw that what he thought was absolutely impossible was really happening: he was walking on water, right through that threatening storm. But as soon as he looked away and focused on the storm, he immediately lost faith (lost "sight") in what God was actually doing for him, and he started sinking again. But when he grabbed hold of Jesus' outstretched hand and kept him in the middle of his vision, his problems faded and he was no longer sinking in desperation. Like us, Peter only had to ask God for help with simple words of desperation, "Lord, save me!" and keep his focus on Jesus, even if he did not understand how this was happening. Then, he quickly saw that things became calm and peaceful, tranquil, and he quickly made it to the other side with Jesus. (Matthew 14:24-33; John 6:16-21) The same things continues to be true for us, too.

This attitude and approach to our problems does not feel natural for us to do, even though we were actually created for it. Like an undeveloped physique which in reality has the same number of muscles as that of any strongman, but is simply out of shape due to lack of using them, it takes exercise to develop the spiritual muscles of our minds. It takes asking God in prayer—an internal sacrifice of surrender and trust—and constant practice...no matter how often we fail along the way. Just like every other athlete does, as well as every other contender for a goal. Suffering is the other side of *passion*: When we truly and deeply love someone more than anything, when we feel passionate about them, we gladly give of ourselves for them. The same goes for any goal that we are passionate about: We are willing to put in the effort and persevere—to continue the struggle—in order to move toward that goal *because it is worth it!* We will not do this perfectly and we will fail often, especially at first; but we *will* grow better through perseverance. When we fall, we keep getting up. Always. That's what counts: The goal is not perfection, but practice. And the sooner we start, the better for us; it's never, ever, too late.

Our heavenly Father will always accept us and never abandon us. He created us for Himself and will turn over heaven and earth for us—we mean that much to Him. In fact, He *will* make something wonderful, positive, and unexpected come out from even our worst cases. He alone will do what we cannot see and what we consider most unlikely. Our job is to *TRUST* Him and keep putting one foot in front of the other. Besides, that's all we really can do. God blesses us beyond our present comprehension through our suffering, our struggles, *with* Him. He uses our adversity to bring impossible good and joy for us, as well as to grow us to become stronger and more resilient, to become more like He is. Let us not lose out on these opportunities by our self-centered thoughts and desires to act out. Let us no longer act like babies; let's let God grow us into the MEN He has created us to be. He *will* make that possible, because that is what He does.

Courageous Man

It takes a man to fight the fight. It is easier to do when we feel strong and that we are winning. But it takes a real man to get up and keep going when he has been knocked down, repeatedly. It takes some courage and strength to get in the ring. It takes the most courage to stay in the ring when we feel weak and scared and not enough. Being a "man" (the ancient Greek word is "andreia") means to keep putting one foot in front of the other, especially when we feel that we don't have what it takes to be alright. This feeling of doubt is normal and natural for us, as is often the case with athletes and other "strugglers." This is where we are authentically human: to admit to ourselves and be willing to accept that, truly, we are not enough. This is how we were intentionally made in our nature, so that we can invite God in to work through us in the struggle and desperation of our daily lives. Life will not necessarily get easier, but it will definitely become more "*do-able*."

We are made in God's image and likeness. Our perfect fit is God alone. We can't do it by ourselves—we will end up defeating our own selves (our minds and spirits by themselves are too weak). News flash: We were not made for ourselves. We have a heart at our core—made in God's image—that can only be filled by inviting God in. This is "cour-age" (from the French word for heart, "coeur"). And being a matter of the heart (the "core" of our nature), this requires faith.

We therefore also need each other: We were made for each other in God's likeness to "en-courage" one another and help one another along. God fills us through each other. God created man and then rested—He now works through *us* as His hands and feet. The soul reflects God, and when one soul connects with another they can complement and center each other.

Concerning our despair when we think ourselves a failure, a holy spiritual father gave this counsel: Never, ever, despair of hope when you fall into sin (that is, when you have a low esteem of yourself); rather, have *courage* and hope in the boundless mercy of God—repent and confess, and you will be saved! In other words, from his deep knowledge and experience of God, he is encouraging the rest of us never to give in to the illusion of hopelessness, but instead to accept the reality of our manhood and God's love: that is, to have courage and take the next step.

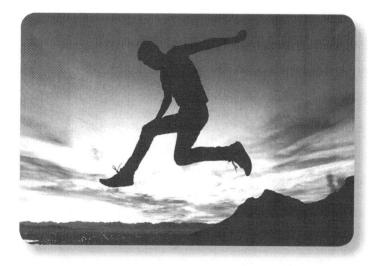

When I Feel Defeated

When I feel down and smashed,
  When I feel crushed and defeated,
    When I feel weak, less-than, a total failure of a man,
      When I feel I am going out of my mind and cry
      out to God in hopeless desperation, "***Oh my dear
      God, why have you abandoned me?!***" ...
Let me remember him who today gave up his everything for
me out of unimaginable love and yearning for me:
  He was threatened with death but did not run and hide,
    He was tortured to death—physically, mentally,
    emotionally—but did not resist,
      He was left alone by his closest friends but did not
      complain,
        He suffered emotionally, mentally, and physically
        to the point of death in Gethsemane, but he did not
        run or medicate,
          He was exposed naked in public with the
          accusation that he acted as if he were a god and
          king, but he did not try to justify himself,
            He was impaled on a tree to die like a total
            loser with other outcast criminals but did not
            defend himself,
            He watched them take all his belongings but
            did not protest,

He was jeered and insulted by all the bystanders, and even by his co-sufferers, but did not try to quiet them,

He watched his mother's heart break to pieces but did not retreat,

He was given sour vinegar to quench his painful thirst but did not comfort himself,

He cried out in my place, "*Eyli, Eyli, lamma shavaqtani?!*" but endured it to his death ...

...So that I will NEVER go through this.

He who is pure and innocent traded places with me once and for all,

So that I, instead, will have the life that *he* deserves.

Yes, that is crazier and far beyond anything I can ever go through...or imagine.

Fulfillment

Like Adam, I was created from the elements of the earth. The word "Adam" is believed to be related to an ancient word for earth or ground, implying a ruddy (reddish) color like the color of clay...and the color of blood and one who has "rosy cheeks." Adam, therefore, implies "from the earth." God breathed life into me and I became a *living soul*. Without connection to Him, I have no life or meaning. My only option is to manufacture an illusion: that my life and existence is worth something only if I meet certain standards. But this is purely an invention of the mind, with no basis in the reality of how I was—and am—created. This mindset then becomes subject to all sorts of lies, influences, and "rationalizations." The inevitable result of this delusion is that I am never perfect, that I am never right or righteous enough. Since I was created with a soul that by its nature always reaches up to something more—to God—I cannot live with the insane lie. So I resort to all sorts of absurd and desperate actions; or I seek to flee or medicate in some way. But I always come back to what is at the center of my very being: my connection with my creator God. I can either try other ways that will only provide a temporary "illusion" of satisfaction but ultimately will make matters worse; or...I can seek to surrender all to Him in simple acceptance and trust—FAITH! "*The **righteous** will live by **faith**.*" (Romans 1:17; Galatians 3:11)

Yearnings

We yearn for and crave (dare I say *lust?*) after God with all our being, as He does for us. He created us for the most intimate heavenly communion with Him. That truth is made real for me through a persevering faith. And I can be with God in all I do, and with everyone.

Because of my weak faith, however, I usually settle for the "created" that I can see, instead of my Creator; I settle for *illusionary* affections and stories, instead of the real. The others can neither fulfill or last, but only deceive and hurt.

All I need is FAITH. That gives courage and assurance. God is real. His Son Jesus, my Christ, is real. His redeeming blood is real. (It is recorded in history forever.) He loves me that much!

Surrender and See God

How can I accept God's love and truly surrender to His truth? The simplest and most direct way I know, which I have learned from wise and blessed men, is to speak directly and plainly with Him. Recognizing that He is truly the core of my essence and loves and desires me beyond all measure (as He does each of us, in a very real, unique, and personal way), I become willing to surrender *my own* notions about God, about myself, about my relationship with Him, about my relationship with others, ...about my whole life. Then, humbly with trust and without fear I confess to Him my sins and my state, and I become willing to accept His unconditional and perfect love for me. More specifically, I do the following "enlightening" exercise as I have learned it from a friend and mentor, and it will work immediately for you, too:

Being willing to except that nothing can change God's love, esteem, and desire for each of us, I lean in with courage (regardless of how much fear and uncertainty I feel) and I ask Him to "forgive me my pride" of that moment. Then, I ask Him to show me how I really see myself; I hold that image for a brief moment. Once more asking Him to forgive my pride, I now ask Him lovingly and with contrition to show me how *He Himself* sees me; again, I hold that image

59

in my mind and heart. Here is what it looks (and sounds) like for me:

1. "Lord, forgive me my sin of pride."
2. "Show me how *I* see myself."
3. "Lord, forgive me again my sin of pride."
4. "Show me how *you* see me through *your* eyes." (And I hold that image!)

Try it. Now. It's that simple...and profound—just as Jesus, I believe, would want it. We reinforce our faith in His truth, love, and unifying redemption by continually doing this. As a further gift and bonus, we also begin humbly (that is, honestly) conversing with Him—as with our closest and most trusted confidant who would never judge us—throughout all our day and in all our tasks. This is what the blessed brother Lawrence of old calls "practicing the presence of God." We carry this over into all our connections and relationships, asking God to be with us and our company, and always giving Him thanks and worship (however simple inside our hearts).

As essentially creatures of relationships and with an infinite (undefinable) psyche, we both seek and promote this real presence of God and the reality of our eternal redemption and "perfected-ness" every time we fellowship with others. And we do so with encouragement, love, and the greatest optimism. Nothing is impossible for our great God(!), and we strengthen ourselves by encouraging one another. We spread the Good News directly and effectively, by just letting God touch the other person through our spirit—and He will do that. That is because the experience and reality and faith and hope of the living God that dwells in our *own* soul can also be received by the *other* soul, through us. We are creatures with souls; we therefore were made for this direct communion with God and with each other. The New Covenant (the new Kingdom, the new "reality") is alive in us! Our Creator God has most realistically redeemed us and perfected us and re-united us to Him through His Son Jesus Christ, through whom we were created in the first place! It is our new reality! Glory to God!

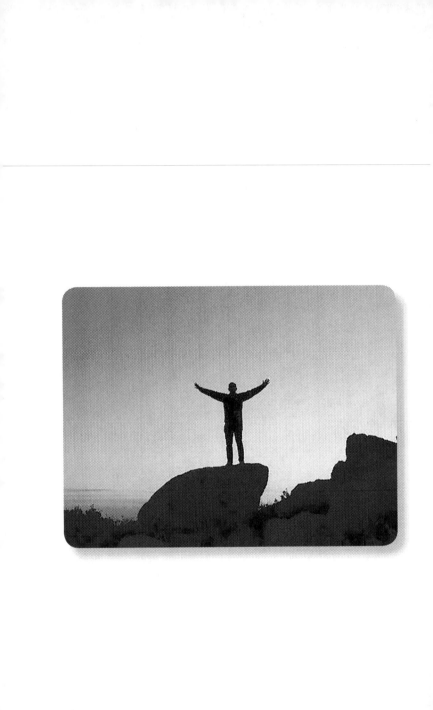

Heartbreak...and Celebration

It breaks God's heart more than anything when we cannot accept His message of outpouring Love, and we reject His longing embrace. Not only has He created us personally for Himself, but He also has paid a very heavy and dear price for it—He has made the ultimate sacrifice for each of us individually, so that we would accept His love and let Him embrace us unconditionally.

But He and *ALL* heaven rejoice in a big and awesome celebration when we DO accept it. ...And in each moment that we do so. (Luke 15:7) How does it feel to know that God and all heaven are celebrating you—yes, *you?* Whether we realize it or not, we *are* that extraordinary in the eyes of our Maker. ...No matter what our current circumstances. So let's take heart and act like it. Because He has already shown to us that we are worth it. Not only that, but we can also be certain that the best is yet to come for us!

Running Backwards

We keep running back to our secret places of deepest shame...
because we feel that we are not worth anything better.

How do we make the message of God's unconditional love
REAL in our lives? Especially when our own faith is not
strong enough; when we are constitutionally too weak; when
the messages from all around us, near and far, tell us that we
are not enough and that we must do the humanly impossible
and be masters of our own destiny?

That's why we need to do works that will encourage us
and one another *with the Truth:* that we ARE loved
unconditionally; that we matter more than *anything else.*
God gave up everything so that we could have His Cross as
a physical reminder of this indisputable Truth.

I'm grateful for my brothers, known and unknown to me, who
are there to encourage me never to forget this and never to
give in to the self-defeating lies that I am alone, a failure, and
that I don't have what it takes to be a success. God put us here
for one another, to encourage each other side-by-side to keep
stepping out forward in the Truth, together as an undefeatable
force—and with the *guarantee* of success already there.

Man's Core, God's Rest

How do we connect with God? How do we tear down those lifelong walls which are based on lies, behind which our irrational fears and insecurities hide? How do we love our neighbor, as Jesus commanded, and have God living in us? How can I accept God's love, when I can't accept myself as being good enough the way that I am? How can I love another brother or sister, when I don't believe that I myself am lovable or right, and when I take this out against my brothers and express it in all that I do? How do I reject the fundamental lie that I am not enough and leave it at the foot of the tree of "knowledge of good and evil" (my tree of "judgement"), and instead except the truth of the Tree of Life that confirms I am perfectly loved and enough exactly as I am?

I don't naturally love my brothers, because there is something wrong at my innermost core—the story that I tell myself about myself. Since I feel so imperfect, I erroneously conclude that I am not good enough and am therefore rejected by God. ...Especially if I've been told that since my childhood, or if that's what I've always been telling myself when I've compared myself to others. But this goes against my very nature, created to live symbiotically (together in harmony) with God...and in His truth that shouts out, "I was made in His image, and therefore I *am* perfectly loved."

And since God is truth, when I don't accept this about myself I am not living in truth. So, I have been living my life all along based on a *lie* about myself. I therefore desperately and irrationally conclude that my only option is to prove myself worthy and good enough to others, on my own, through my own abilities, achievements, and power. This is in order to gain approval and acceptance and have "creds" among those around me (and especially inside my own head)—as if that were enough to fill my core, which I mistakenly believe is rotten or empty. As a result, I cannot see God's presence which is already dwelling (built-in) inside of me, at my very core—the truth, as He created me.

The lie about myself is at the fundamental core of my awareness. And as I go through my daily life with my thoughts, observations, and interactions with others and with my environment, this false story is being reinforced constantly. That is because this false *illusion* and its accompanying feelings lead me to continuously draw the same erroneous conclusions about myself. Therefore, it drives or influences from the deepest level all of my motivations—without exception—both internally and externally: It is at the core of how I think and how I behave.

If I cannot accept myself in truth as being good enough and right, then I am not able to love my neighbor: I cannot believe in God's love for me, so how can I pass on true love to others? All of my actions and attention naturally become self-serving, and I don't even realize it. Moreover, nothing I can do can ever change my faulty perception about myself, especially when I see my many faults and shortcomings. But the truth is that all of my achievements, as well as all of my faults, don't change the person I really am in my soul and core: The created cannot change its nature without the Creator. How I see myself, however, *can* change. That is where grace comes in.

Since God actually expressed His personal love for me so completely through Jesus Christ within my very own physical and human existence (that is, in actual human history), I can humbly accept this gift and God's love for me and at last become willing to give up all of my own conclusions and expectations. (Think about that again.) I can finally live and breathe this "true reality" more and more naturally as I ask for God's help constantly and practice being consciously aware of his presence within me, no matter how often I get distracted or fall—this may be frequent at first, but the point is to keep getting up and continuing with it: I invite Him in and talk to Him (just as I would to a trusted friend). All the time, as often as I can remember to do it. I am now letting Him work in me to tear down my walls and faulty vision about myself built by so many years of lies. When I can accept myself as I am (just as God does), when I can accept God's love for me through Jesus Christ and his redeeming and loving atonement for me, then I can accept and love my neighbor in truth (without condition). No more poisonous attitudes for me! I can therefore experience God's love by giving it and letting it be expressed through me. God lives inside of me, and I now believe it!

This truth and life, of course, is also reflected in every aspect of my existence: physically, emotionally, mentally, and spiritually. God's love is not expressed just on my inside— it is also acted out in all my relationships. This is sanity and wholeness. It is only made possible through faith in Jesus

Christ (that is, belief in the Truth: God's love for me). He is our healer and savior (Amen!), and my faith and acceptance of this truth frees me from the obstructive lies, and in their place flows the gift of grace.

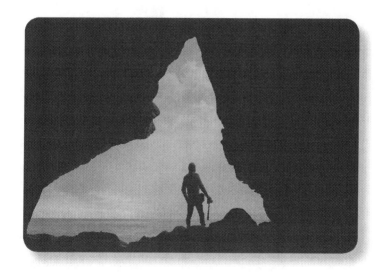

Greatest Sorrow

It must grieve God to no end when we reject His passionate love for us—His undying yearning for deepest intimacy with us. Just look at what He has sacrificed to attract us and have us! He gave up not only Himself fully, but even his most beloved and only child…His *only* Son. God has proven to us that He loves us even more than His own self, even more than everything else precious to Him. He created us to *live* intimately with us in every second of every day. To do His will *through* us so that we share in His glory—He loves us that much!

God often reaches out and He Himself personally touches us through other people in whom He dwells. They, too, want to share this experience in communion with us. All too often, however, because of our fears and hurts and the false stories we believe about ourselves, we keep these people and their message at a distance, not wanting to let anyone inside where they could see the "real" us. So, without ever admitting it to ourselves or others, we really think that low of ourselves! The truth, however, is that this is completely opposite of the real way that God sees us and feels about us. When we reject God in the people He sends to us, we deeply hurt these "angels," and we grieve God's Spirit beyond understanding…because He completely desires us that much, and He has gone to the extreme to make Himself available to us personally, as if we ourselves were the only people in the world for Him.

So, how do we develop an attitude of constantly inviting God in? We pray for it, and we practice...a lot, constantly. When we forget or are distracted throughout the day, we don't get frustrated; we just remind ourselves of God's presence and do it: We *talk* to Him, as honestly and openly as we would talk to our greatest confidante and biggest admirer. We involve Him in everything and share everything with Him: our joy, our gratitude, our fears, our weaknesses, our anger, our (secret) desires, what we think about ourselves— especially those things we want to hide from God and others. And especially our deepest wounds and our deepest secrets: those things that we want to take to our graves and of which we are most ashamed. Don't worry, everybody has them, and God has heard it all many times before; He understands our heart and never judges us or condemns us. Besides, He already knows it and wants to free us of their burden when we are willing to admit them to Him, willing to *let go* of them. For a long time, we have hidden these in the deepest crevices of our soul—right where God wants to be. In fact, that's where we've suppressed the reflection of His image (in which we were created; our *true selves*) and instead replaced it with the illusion that we are "unsatisfactory" and unacceptable. As a result, these false stories are now buried at our inner core and have become the deepest foundation that is driving our motivations, feelings, and attitudes... about ourselves, others, and even about God.

If we do not become willing to look at and remove these core falsehoods by surrendering them to God, we will continue to live by the lies of our own stories about ourselves. Wise people with much personal experience through the ages have reminded us that we are "as sick as our secrets." We constantly try to compensate on the outside for what we feel are deficiencies on our inside. We also try to run away from and medicate our feelings of inadequacy. We can't live with this sense of being "wrong," so we often take it out on other people (especially those closest to us). Often, we are not even aware that we are doing this—we've convinced ourselves that is obviously someone else's fault that we feel so bad. None of our attempts to "cope" work, and our irrational desperation only grows more intense and drives us to seek external fulfillments, compensations, and "fixes." We may even try to fill this "God-sized" hole in us with relationships that we have no right to. We squander our birth-right as royal children of God who are free, and we instead give ourselves to others and become dependent upon them to make us feel right and complete. In essence, we become enslaved. But we ultimately find that nothing and nobody can make us feel "whole," and we are soon disappointed; then we try again with even greater desperation to grasp on to other things and people. As we continue in this downward spiral, we bring down those around us and destroy our healthy relationships, our ability to make sound judgments, and even our sense of purpose and self-worth. ...Until we get to the blessed point of finally becoming open to learn and accept another way.

We become open to help by whatever means it takes. We invite God into these areas, tell Him how it makes us feel, and talk to him most honestly about it. We don't worry about how we think He may judge us—He already knows our brokenness and yearns to heal us. We invite Him in there and share it openly with Him. We put aside our own sense of pride and our own judgments about right and wrong, and for once we open up completely to God in the most intimate, honest, and authentic way. We become willing to show God who and what we really think we are on the inside. ...And then we ask Him to show us how *He* sees us. We ask Him to heal us with His *truth* about us. And He does just that, out of the unimaginable love and desire and purpose that He has for us. He has already proven that to us as a guarantee.

It's simple: Being fulfilled is about accepting God's love for us...in everything we do, in everything we are, and in everything we experience. Then we are really free from our misconceptions and we are living in reality.

Key to Freedom from Sin

Just a thought to share with my brothers: The key to freedom from sin is...faith and trust that God has already taken care of it and redeemed me. I therefore surrender and let go of my self-judgment and self-condemnation. Whenever it rears its ugly head, I picture myself giving it over to God. A friend once shared with me this visual technique of letting go of such thoughts: Whatever my problem is, I picture that I am holding it in the form of a long cloth (like a tablecloth), and then I drape it over my image of God; and I watch it disappear. That quick and simple exercise helps me let go of it from my mind, and it can be done easily anywhere, anytime.

Unfortunately, I've wasted most of my (Christian) life not believing and truly accepting in my core that God loves me no matter what and never judges me or condemns me. What a gross shame and waste for me!

Saint Paul explains it: "*All* have sinned and fall short of the glory of God, being *justified freely* by His grace through the redemption that is in Christ Jesus." (Romans 3:23-24; bold and italic enhancement made here for emphasis.) That means His justification from any condemnation applies to you and me 100% no matter what. All we have to do is *believe* it. And again: "And having been set free from sin, you became slaves of righteousness." (Romans 6:18) The term "slaves of righteousness" means that we are forever bound to the *freedom of righteousness*, that we are forever free of guilt—and free of judgment and condemnation—in Jesus Christ. With that freedom comes our responsibility to act like it: *I no longer have the right to judge myself,* nor to run and medicate and take my bad feelings out on others. Instead, I accept my God-given and permanent status as a righteous man, and I just do the next right thing. Think about it: If God has justified me and freed me, who then can ever condemn me? (Romans 8:31-34)

This freedom from sin, of course, doesn't mean I will always overcome temptations and that I will no longer sin; I am still a weak human. Rather, by Jesus' redemption (effective through my repentance, faith, and trust), my sin is pardoned and no longer counts against me; that is, it no longer has a slave-hold on me to condemn me. (Romans 5:1-2) So, then, why shouldn't I simply continue to do those "sinful" things that I like to do…since I can always repent afterwards, and since God will always forgive me and never condemn me? The better question is: Why would I willingly go back to doing those things that hurt me and others and that make me hate—especially *myself*—all over again? (Romans 6:21) The point is that in my new journey of freedom and self-respect, I need only focus on taking the next right step; I may continue to fall short at times and to sin and suffer against my better judgment, but God no longer judges me. If only I, too, could always do the same (that is, not judge myself). If only I had more trust—I would be a happier man, knowing that I am always free.

Perhaps this daily struggle is another way of "suffering for Christ," suffering to accept his truth about me. It is this truth that sets me free! All I have to do is believe it; and if I have trouble doing so, I still act like it and ask God for help to accept it. (Mark 9:24) It will become more natural in just a short time. God makes this possible. ...Because that it is His explicit will for me, which He continues to demonstrate over and over again in my life—after all, I am still here. That means that God is waiting for me to accept His liberating truth about me, and for me to live the way He always intended for me: as a ***truly free man***, free of any judgment and never condemned!

<u>Note</u>: *For more on this, see for yourself how well Saint Paul wrote about this key subject in his letter to the Romans, chapters 3-8.*

Desires

All of my desires have their origin and goal in God. It may sound absurd at first, but it is actually logical and only natural to be that way. Here's why: I was created with a soul—a psyche, a mind of spirit (the core driver of my wants and will)—that naturally yearns to reach and connect with something outside of myself, something bigger than myself: something *more* to "satisfy" me and give me rest and a sense of comfort within myself. This is often desired and sought for in relationships with people, in objects, and in achievements, whether actual or theoretical (merely how it seems to be in my own mind). At the most basic level, I am yearning and searching for something to give me a personal, internal, sense of being enough… of being whole and "right." Since this involves my inner self, my *soul*—and since the soul understands, responds to, and thrives on *relationships*— my deepest sense of desire can feel satisfied through my connections, through my honest and intimate relationships: where soul meets soul, where we connect with God through someone in His image and likeness. As wonderful and necessary as these are, and as totally gratifying as they can feel at first, none of these people, objects, and achieved goals can be—solely by themselves—a sufficient substitute for connection with the *real* God Who is without limit, restriction, or shortcoming…for the One I am really looking for deep down. Therefore, even with my bucket list (as well as my "secret" hidden list) all checked off, I will always be searching for more. And since I am human—with a physical body, chemistry, and emotions—my desires become ever more complicated, and my ways to satisfy them become ever more creative. Obsessions take over, and then habits and addictions become hard to beat and lead to more and more trouble.

My only true solution is to surrender *all* of my desires (especially the secret ones) and my will to God, and to seek rest and complete satisfaction in Him only. Of course, that doesn't mean giving up my other wants, needs, and relationship—just putting *God* first. It seems like a very difficult concept at the outset, and even one that is impossible: to put God as my true heart's desire and goal *above* all my loved ones, all my wants, and all my personal aspirations. It may even seem like something that sounds nice to certain religious people but is just a "philosophical" and abstract idea, something that is not practical and "practice-able" in the everyday life of a man like me; something that is not even *necessary*, to be blunt and honest. Why can't I keep my life and wants and desires and my personal world separate from the "God" stuff? Simply put, because I will more than likely end up making a mess of things for myself and others (since I don't know everything and I am not all-powerful), and I will surely end up losing everything that I have put in God's place—in the place of my deepest "desire." That's just the way it is, the way I was created…and it's actually a gift beyond all my understanding and greater than any and all desires I may now have or even dream about. Putting God first will allow me to enjoy my relationships and all I have in a much, much deeper and fulfilling way. That is because I have an immaterial and immortal soul (one that by nature seeks something more than itself), which means I was created by a spiritual God in *His* image and likeness, and which means that He made me for *Himself* and for a real purpose: to share life with Him, to share in His everyday miracles with Him, to relate to and touch other souls with Him, to enjoy all pleasures in Him... In short, to be His conduit in this material, human world where there are other beings with a soul just like me. This business is not about my having to give up all people and things that are important to me and that I desire—that would seem cruel and unrealistic. Rather, it is about *priorities:* putting God first by trusting that He knows best and that He loves me more than anything, and therefore *entrusting* everyone and everything I love and desire to Him and to His will. Nothing makes God happier than to invite Him in to be with—and work through—me! That's why He created me, with a soul, in the first place.

In reality and in everyday living, this is not only very doable, but also very simple in nature; after all, that's how I was created. All I have to do is make a start, even a very small one. That's all. Then, the wheels of progress start moving, guaranteed. This is what surrender looks like to me: When I'm about to start anything, or when I feel myself "wanting" something in someway, I tell God that I am giving it to Him. I tell Him that I trust He will see that I get what is absolutely best for me...and best for His Kingdom. I don't even have to completely believe it—I just have to be *willing* to accept it, and then do the next right thing (even if that means I don't take any action at the moment). This way, I am participating with God's perfect and unstoppable will; I'm not merely trying to figure things out on my own and put things together in a haphazard manner. Moreover, I am not doing anything *alone* anymore. I no longer expect myself (count only on myself) to make things, people, and circumstances be a certain way, the way *I* think they should be—I have always failed at that, and I've frustrated myself (and those around me) to no end trying to make it "be" my way. I no longer have the attitude that it is all up to me. Even if I were all-powerful, I still do not know everything in order to ensure that the best turns out. So, I realize that my old way of thinking has been not only impractical, but also ridiculous. How much time and energy I have wasted trying to live that way; and how many people I have hurt, especially myself and those closest to me. Some wise people have summarized the new way of living this way: Simply do the next right thing and leave the consequences to God; however it turns out is the way it's supposed to be. It may sound too simple for a complicated person like me, but it is nevertheless true. Jesus did not come to complicate our lives, but to free us from the complications of life. He urges us lovingly and with surety to trust God just like little children, with simplicity and innocence. That attitude opens my mind to live life from God's perspective. (Luke 18:16-17)

This way of thinking and daily living seems contrary to what I've always learned—and what others have stressed to me—about *becoming* successful and making "something" of myself in order to be judged as right and supposedly feel satisfied, fulfilled and happy in my life. So this new attitude will not *feel* natural to me at first. No problem: I simply go to God with this continuously, as often as I can remember, and ask for his help and grace. Specifically, I ask Him to help me love Him and trust Him, and I let Him do the rest. I don't let myself get discouraged when I feel I can't keep up this "surrender of desires," or when I think it is useless for me. Instead, like the man that I am and like every other athlete, I just get up and keep putting one foot in front of the other. That's all I have to do. The amazing thing is that I CAN'T LOSE, no matter how often I fall, forget, or seem to fail... Because I am not doing this on my own. With each passing day, this becomes easier and more natural—just like doing anything new. I soon see (for real!) that with my own self-centered and imperfect expectations out of the way, I've actually opened the channel and invited God to give me wonderful fulfillment and joy in my relationships and strivings, and with everything I get. When I surrender these to Him, He sets me free to enjoy them boundlessly, like a small child. As the blessed St. Augustine said, after much restlessness, troubles, and heartache, "Oh Lord, You have made us for Yourself, and our heart is restless until it finds its rest in You!"

A revealing footnote:

> We covet and desire only what we think we don't have. When I deny that I have a certain quality in myself (such as being "enough", being "desirable"), I naturally lust after it. I lust to get from others what I don't accept is true about myself. But the reality is, I already have it—I just can't see it in myself. This denial misleads me to see myself as incomplete, and the desperation drives me to try to get it from other places. That's why it can never satisfy: because it's not *reality*.

> What *is* real is that I already have "it" (the quality of being enough) through Jesus

Christ, through whom I was created in God's image as a unique and *complete* man, and redeemed of any shortcomings (and of any *ideas* of shortcomings) by his very blood. He took on *my* personal nature, and therefore shares with me *his* nature of Truth. We are one with the only truth: Jesus, you, and I together. (John 17:20-23) There is no judgment about myself or others, because there is no difference in Christ. We are a new, *full* creation. We are perfected in Jesus Christ. That is the message, the "good news," that is explained and blasted aloud in the Gospels and urgently declared by countless people throughout the ages.

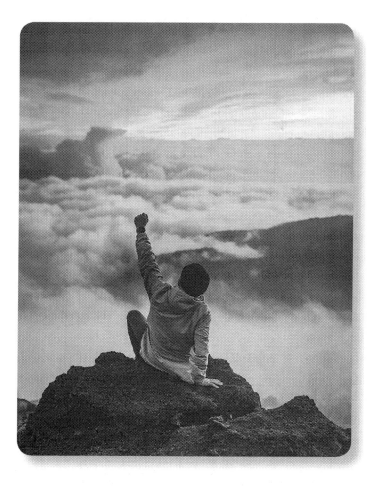

The Answer

My mind is constantly seeking a state of comfort, peace, and tranquility—a sense of being "right." That is only natural, because God created me with a soul that yearns to connect with something higher, something perfect. However, this cannot be achieved by human laws or standards. That has proven to be the case throughout all of human history...and in my own life.

The answer is my Creator, the Logos (that is, the "Word"), the son of God, Jesus Christ—through whom I and all things were created. There is nothing I can do to satisfy myself as being right and comfortable. It is just a temporary illusion, a lie not based on absolute Truth and reality. The idea that I am enough, perfect, righteous is only made real in believing in the "redemption" of Jesus Christ. This means that *he* has done something for me that I cannot make happen for myself. He has paid for all my shortcomings, and I am perfected in him. The Creator Word of God who has made me in his image has made right all my shortcomings; or rather, he makes me be right in spite of my shortcomings, so that they no longer count against me.

Because this is a matter of the inner man—the eternal and absolute essence of my being—it is a *spiritual* matter. Therefore, this is made real and alive in me through *faith*.

And faith opens me up to receive guaranteed grace. To have faith means the Word lives in me and I in him. The "answer" is: I am complete and perfect in him. He prefers only to live in me and I in him! This man (you, me) now is one with God—forever! Praise and glory be to God forever! And His great power and love and work is beyond all understanding. That's why it takes more than my mind—it takes faith! Faith is not just a matter in the mind. It is ALIVE—it brings life. Therefore, God is the *meaning* of my life, and this has been made possible through his Word Jesus Christ in the Holy Spirit. All it requires of me for this to become my reality is acceptance in faith: Faith, therefore, brings meaning and reality into my life—I am truly alive through faith!

The Message—The Experience

The Bible is the story of man, of each one of us. It's the story of our *own* lives. As humans, we are eternal souls in a worldly existence. We all share a common experience. We all share the same experiences to one degree or another. The Bible captures many facets of our common human reality. It shows over and over how much our God and Creator loves us and is faithful to us. …To *us,* whom He created in His own image and redeemed with a price that cost Him more than His own self: the life of His only child. He did that out of His unimaginable love and concern for you and me, His "human" and very real children. The scriptures are written so that we can all relate to every story and experience in the Bible in our own unique ways. Just like a loving father relates to each of his children in their own special way, with no two relationships exactly the same but tailored to meet the individual, unique child right where they are.

The message is God's love and living word to us. It is more than just human words to be processed and evaluated by our brain. Because of the nature of our soul—made for, and yearning for, a connection with its higher Creator—we can connect to this message with our very soul. That is where the transformation happens. That is why the good news and message is best related personally, from one person to another, from one soul to another—the Spirit lives and moves in the soul and gives life. Just like it is happening here. It concerns people who are like you and me. It is not meant to be simply a story or book for reading and meditation and learning. It is written, rather, to inspire, to invigorate, and to *transform us.* (John 6:63) It does so through the eternal truth of its message that is conveyed in human terms through human experiences of people like us...with our human DNA. (Yes, each of us was in the DNA of our first forefather— Adam, if you will.) Like God Himself, His message is not merely an object—it is a human *experience* that is relevant to all of us. ...A personal love-letter from God Himself to each of us. And it is saying that a very special Someone (your Creator, God Himself) is madly in love with you.

Freedom

Being a child of God means that I have been set free from sin. It means that sin is no longer a condemning sentence for me, as Saint John reminds us throughout his first letter (1 John 1:7, 3:5, 3:9). I may still stumble into it and suffer from it, but it no longer has the power to hold me and condemn me; nor to *define* me. Transgression of the law no longer binds me to sin; the debt has been paid by the son of God Jesus, forever! (Romans 6:3-11, 8:1-4)

The sneaky lie that tries to convince me that I must perform well in order to be right or righteous is smashed and vanishes like smoke. I am no longer bound under the law. And that is by the grace of the redemption of Jesus Christ, which is made effective and real in my life through my faith. Just as faith was reckoned to holy Abraham as righteousness (Genesis 15:6; Romans 4:3).

The power of the law has been broken. The power of the lie that we must meet certain "standards" in order to be right, is deflated and neutralized. You and I are truly *free!*

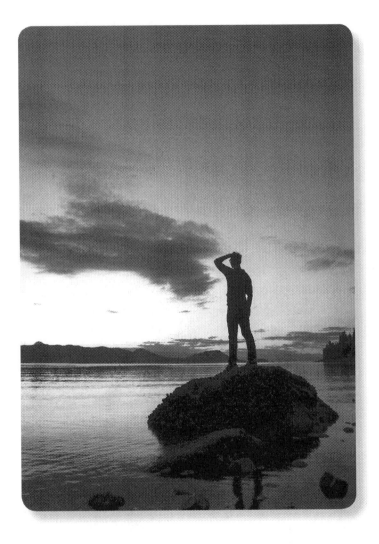

No More Sin

Christ's redemption has freed us from the power of sin and judgment. In Christ, through faith, we are no longer slaves to sin and judgment. "Go, and sin no more," says Jesus many times throughout the Gospels, specifically after healings. But what does this actually mean? What does it look like in practical terms? Besides, who can actually do this (never sin again), and how is this even possible for a human being, especially one like me? This *is* possible when we look at from another way, from the *truth* (*God's* truth): we are *already* perfect in him (Jesus the Christ) through grace. And this is made "real" in our lives and actually applies to us through *faith* (this will be explained just below). Of course, this does not mean that we will never do anything wrong again. On the contrary, we are human and God is the only one Who is sinless. So it is God Who is doing this in us, through Christ who has already paid for and nullified any condemnation for our sins. Yes, we are prone to sin in this world, and we along with everyone suffers from it— even the saints sinned... every day. But God (the only Judge) keeps us "perfect" in His eyes by grace, that is, for free, out of unconditional love for us no matter what we do. (Romans5:1-2; Romans 8:35-39) Though we make mistakes and still do wrong at times, we are not "judged" or condemned or sentenced by this. Instead, through our willingness (and courage) to still affirm God's "unconditional" love for us and ask for forgiveness—that is, when we are willing to maintain this *faith*—we enter into the reality where He has removed any mark from us and cleansed us through the blood He already poured out for us forever. In other words, any sentence we deserve has already been paid, and we—by accepting it through faith (or at least, being willing to accept it)—have a clean slate again. In this way, we are indeed "sinless" and free from judgment.

There is a saying that the difference between saints and sinners is that the saints, after they fall into sin, keep getting up and moving forward in their faith. In other words, it's about the decisions we make on that same journey which either lift us into a type of personal Paradise on Earth…or dig our the hole of our mental suffering even deeper.

Christ's holy redemption is real for us in every moment. And we do well to acknowledge this as often as possible, especially when we break bread (every time we eat and take "nourishment"). That is because the enemy of our souls keeps trying to deceive us not to believe the reality of our redemption (our freedom from sin) that God has gone to such pains to prove to us. Since he has no power to take us away from God's love, he tries constantly to deceive us into *thinking* and *feeling* we are not loveable anymore, that we are hopeless sinners, in order to trick us into hiding…from God and from ourselves. We then turn our focus away from God's love by believing the lie that He no longer could want us. So we try harder to take matters into our own hands and make ourselves *seem* desirable and *feel* comfortable. We'll do anything to distract ourselves from the insane desperation produced by the lie that we—our true selves, as we are—no longer matter. Feeling desperate and hopeless, we medicate any way we can, and we try to expunge (remove and transfer) this pain onto others by hurting them, perhaps unconsciously.

We are therefore driven and willing to commit more wrongs, more "sins," to make ourselves feel better and *fix* things for ourselves, out of fear and anger to get what we feel we deserve to have. But in the end, this only feeds the lie in our minds that we are bad, broken, unlovable, undesirable...and hopeless. So the vicious cycle only repeats itself, growing ever worse, and we further hurt ourselves and those close to us. We have let ourselves become "enslaved" by this illusion about our sinfulness: that there is something wrong about us. As a result, sin is our reaction to the lie that we are not right or good enough—just like Adam and Eve believed when tricked by the serpent, while they were actually *in* Paradise and walking with God.

How do we break such a cycle of sin? The hard truth is, we are powerless on our own to make ourselves right. ***God's love*** is the answer and the solution. It's what gives meaning to our lives. He proved it for each one of us, individually, through the very real actions of His Son Jesus Christ. So we have an actual *event* rooted in our history, our existence, our reality, upon which we can pin our hope and faith with conviction. (1 Peter 1:21) And ***faith*** (acceptance of this fact, and acting like we accept it) is what makes this *real* for us: we become willing to believe in God's unconditional love and desire for us and approval of us, brokenness and all. We just accept that we are perfect and enough in His eyes. We don't have to understand it, but only accept what He has *factually* done for us during Jesus' life on Earth. That's what clears away the insanity and replaces the hopeless desperation with deep serenity. We feel fulfilled, valuable and valued, worthy, and, above all, loved. We are not interested in doing wrong to others or to ourselves, because we feel and *know* we are perfect as we are.

A related note: Perhaps the most stealthy and deceptive lie is the one that promotes "false" pride: believing that through our actions—especially those that look like piety or "correct-ness" on the outside—we can somehow make ourselves "right" and acceptable on the inside. Instead, this pride enslaves us in our minds under the "law" of what we *should* be like...and that we can get there on our own merely by doing such-and-such. That negates our faith in and reliance upon grace, which means "*free* gift." It implies that, actually, we do not accept God's unconditional love and acceptance of us ("unconditional" means: as we are, no matter what). And this is where we judge ourselves—and everyone around us—all the more and are further tempted to sin out of desperation, since we deny Christ's freeing (and *free*) redemption and instead try insanely to do the impossible on our own.

To summarize: The biggest lie we tell ourselves is that "... because of my actions I am no longer 'worthy' of God's grace." Nothing could be farther from the Truth. We break that lie by being willing to believe in God's unconditional, *personal* love for us and acceptance of us. It must hurt Him deeply when we reject this truth, which cost Him so dearly to prove to us: the truth that we *are* loved and now sinless in His eyes. We are, in this very real sense, truly free from sin.

The Mystery Journey— Through the Wilderness

Our attempts to cope with our existence and manage our life in this world solely on our own power leads to much frustration and ultimately *profound desperation.* It is exactly through this sense of inadequacy that God, in turn, leads us to his Truth. When we finally realize that we cannot manage life to be the way we want it to be, no matter what we do, only then can we become willing to accept another way besides our own. We become capable of genuinely accepting God's will in our lives only by giving up the place of our old ideas and theories and being open to learn his Truth. And that Truth is that God has everything under control for us and is able (and eager!) to do everything for our good, and that He always loves us unconditionally—no matter what—and sees us as perfect exactly as we are. Specifically, He wants to give us not just what we think we need, but rather exactly what we are most yearning for in the deepest part of our souls: a sense of peace, confident optimism, connection, perfect fulfillment, unshakable hope, and absolute "right-ness."

But surrendering our old ways of thinking about life—that it is up to us to make things turn out right—does not come naturally or easily to us. As it has been said by wise men: We have to become as willing to learn as only the dying can be. On our own, our "psyche"—expressed in our ego, judgments and conclusions, disposition, mind, and will—is naturally weak, imperfect ("sick"), and inadequate. We come to accept the simple reality that by ourselves we are not bigger than the world and this life. Such surrender is true humility, and it most often comes only after suffering the dire consequences of our own "self-ish" ways. But we can also pray that God will open us up to this deep surrender; and He *will* make that possible...because *that* is what He wants most and is His great pleasure to do!

To invite the Almighty in to run our lives, it is necessary to be willing to leave behind our old ways, concepts, views, and expectations. These have always been insufficient for us and the reason for our frustrations and let-downs. With just our "willingness" to surrender, God will make it a reality that will definitely transform us: We just put one foot in front of the other. When God leads us on this journey, we are like sojourners in a foreign land—just like the Bible patriarchs and other holy figures. It means that in a figurative way we leave our "old land and kin" and venture into the unknown wilderness. It is scary and takes the commitment of a real man—that's you and me!—just as it was for all pioneers into a new world. It is on this journey, with all its trials and challenges, that we are transformed through our persevering faith and grace into the reality of the new man: the new Adam with the reality of God's breath as our life. Though we may not see our progress at first, the world and its ways will soon seem different (inadequate) and strange to us...and the world will notice that we, too, are somehow different. We now live in *God's* kingdom, in God's realm (God's "reality"). We are no longer easily disturbed and distracted, or driven by of our fears and desperation. All we have to do is keep going, keep getting back up and moving forward, doing the next right thing. Through our endurance, we will see that the journey itself is our destination, one that grows brighter with every step forward. It will seem like a slow and hard trudge at times, but it will always be doable, and it is exactly the stuff of a true hero's adventure.

After a short time, we see that this is difficult and even impossible to maintain *on our own.* That's why we are dependent on God's grace and our faith. We need the encouragement of the Holy Spirit and, by extension, of each other. We are naturally social creatures who need connection to our Creator—both directly and through each other—as we live in the world. The journey is made more doable when we walk with our brothers. And they are right there next to us, whether we can actually see them or not. Trust your faith. If you are reading this, then know that there are already brothers (co-pioneers, co-warriors) by your side. How awesome and out-of-this-world is that?!

Awakening into Reality—
Dispelling the Delusion

We know from our own human experience that the only reality, the only "absolute" reality, is the *presence of God*. Everything else has to do with our own limited perceptions and subjective imagination of how things are. This imperfect and unsure vision feeds our fears and insecurities, and we are all driven by a desperate desire to feel whole, comfortable, and in control—to feel optimistic about being able to do it... *alone*. After all, we have been constantly told that "it" is up to us and that "we" are the masters of our own destinies. The indisputable truth remains, however, that as spiritual beings with a psyche (a soul with a mind that dreams about bigger things and yearns for a higher connection), we were created by a Higher Being, God Who is beyond this material world, to *live* in true reality and to be alive and free...through eternal and real communion with Him.

The only way I can do this is to sincerely invite God in, by letting go of my own will—my own desires and expectations, my own goals. These are based only on my own concept, my *illusion*. of what will make things right. This God of ours has made every single one of us, personally, for something much bigger and better than that. My own will is based on my incomplete and imperfect (and therefore "faulty") perceptions and conclusions, and the fears and desires that they arouse inside of me. These can often be traced back to very early experiences and the conclusions I had drawn from them at the time. Consequently, these old experiences and the faulty conclusions I had made (based on the terror and pain I had felt at that time) continue to control me like a terrifying bully, and I am kept bound ("enslaved") to that deep-rooted thought process and the automatic reactions that persist inside of me. These may be just ideas that continue inside my head, but their effects are overpowering and very real in my body and mind. They are truly a big deal that affects both my life and those around me, and it is so worth the effort to get the healing and restoration that I need (I am not stronger than my own mind). Although I have a mind and a soul that naturally seeks to reach beyond itself, I cannot fully understand or manufacture my right (sound, healthy) reality on my own. So, how do I get there? And what can I do to get healed from my deep-seated notions and reactions? Besides any professional or other special help I may need, is there anything further that I can do for myself to be free of, to "surrender," my old ways, my defective will?

Practicing the *presence of God* habitually and in all things— as much as is possible for me at the time—is the quickest way I know to surrender my will. The good news is that it doesn't mean I have to change who I am or become a "living saint" or super-religious person. ...Nor a far-out spiritualist. I can just be myself, exactly where I am now—that's all I *can* be, in all honesty. And that's where God delights to meet me. We have the example and collected words of the blessed brother Lawrence (compiled in the work "The Practice of the Presence of God") to help us do this "simple" but transforming exercise. (More about this below.) I also keep in mind that my *own* will, even when it is well intentioned, is fundamentally motivated by my sense of "ego": how I *myself* see things, and my desire to make things right on my own. Sometimes this appears to be helpful, but it is always lacking in wisdom and ultimately proves to be not enough...

As hard as it is to accept, we all are like passengers aboard the Titanic: none of us will get off this planet alive (a famous bumper-sticker saying). We can try to maintain the illusion that the end is not a reality for *us* aboard our Titanic, and we can try to keep at bay the increasingly desperate, albeit quiet, voice inside of us by distracting ourselves with rearranging the deck-chairs and making plans to attend the fun and grand shipboard events. Often—this is a favorite "escape"— we imagine in our minds situations and stories which elicit brain chemistry that makes us *feel* really good, just like in a daydream. But sooner or later we will have to face the reality—there is no escaping it. The question, then, is: Do we continue to live in denial, with its inherent delusions and increasingly futile attempts to cope, which only complicate our lives with further problems and bring us to clash with others? Do we continue pretending to know what's going on, what the big picture is and where we fit in it? Do we keep trying to gloss over our feelings of insecurity and uselessness by latching our sense of self-worth and "right-ness" onto other people and things and goals (imagined or real), which could never suffice for us in that way? Do we continue struggling to push away the insane idea that our life is basically meaningless and therefore hopeless? Or... Do we stand with comfort and courage in the assured reality and happy knowledge that everything is actually under control amidst these circumstances, and that our own personal lifeboat is waiting to take us to an even better ship, one that is truly invincible and has nothing but first-class accommodations for all? Will we, therefore, live the rest of our time here on our Titanic knowing that *this* journey was meant to be only temporary; that it is a necessary voyage that gets us to the next one—our permanent and perfect home? Will we live with this awesome reality in our hearts and minds, and even help our fellow passengers wherever and whenever we can? How do I do this?

As long as I am bound by a worldly view and approach to life, my will and actions will inevitably end up imperfect and unsatisfying. In spite of how things appear to *us,* God's perfection and rightness is not the same as what we think it should be in our own limited concepts and understanding. Therefore, we must be willing to take steps to let go of this faulty and inadequate way of thinking and living. And we can actually do this easily anytime and everywhere, inside ourselves in our private space with God. That is where we practice the presence of God, and it aligns our mind and our vision with *His* perfect reality. There is no right way to do it, nor any time requirements—it is perfect as long as we are *honest.* And that's all that God wants from us, because He loves us too much to infringe on our will. He already knows our deepest hurt and fears...they reside in our core, where He is. And it's from there that they have distorted our view of God, His personal love for us, and His reality. But that is also where God is waiting for us to meet Him and heal us, at the place of our deepest problems. A *willingness* to be honest with ourselves—to look at these wounds and talk about them with total honesty—opens the path for us to get there.

So, here we go: We sincerely ask God to help us. ...In spite of the pain, paralyzing fears, ferocious anger, and doubt that we may have. We look at our inner motives and we *talk with God* plainly and honestly in everything we do, as often as we can remember to do it. Just being ourselves to God, with all our honesty. We don't try to act or talk the way *we* think it should be done for God to approve of us. He delights more than anything to be in our honest company, exactly as we are at the moment. Don't worry, you won't offend God; remember, He *wants* us to talk to Him personally and with *complete* honesty, knowing that He *never* judges or condemns us but loves us *unconditionally*. We just do the best we can at this little exercise in our current circumstances, and we don't judge ourselves about it. This will likely mean we have to let go of our restricting image of God and of how we think that He will react to our drop-dead honesty—that view of Him has always been an obstacle to us.

To help me with this last point, I can make a list of qualities that I would want my perfect and loving God to have, if I could have Him be *my* way. (In other words, how I wish God really was.) And I can use *that* for my starting image, while keeping an open mind for something even better than I can imagine right now. Now I won't have to be afraid or too angry to talk about myself and my situation, my thoughts and feelings, my fears and pain and struggles, etc., with my own Creator. I can even tell Him how I feel about doing this. God has demonstrated over and over with countless "real" people all throughout history who were just like you and me (and often much bigger "sinners" than we think of ourselves) that He loves us *unconditionally* and delights to heal us continuously, no matter what. We can therefore begin the inward journey of living in His reality—His presence— one step at a time. Throughout our day as we go about our routine, we constantly examine our motivations with an open mind, willing to reject our own self-made judgments and conclusions. We are mindful of God and "practice" His presence with us by talking to Him and sharing with Him as with a most loyal confidante. We do so as much as we can in all our tasks and actions, no matter how big or small, or how shameful or proud we feel. We also invite God into all our contacts, encounters, and relationships; and we encourage one another through fellowship. We don't obsess over this; we just try to remember to do it as often and as simply as we can—it will become more and more habitual.

This exercise of constant self-examination (definitely *not* self-judgment) and on-going conversations with God will not seem natural to us at first. We will likely think at the beginning that it's not helping or working for us, and we will be tempted to just give up. Perhaps we will think it is too painful and too much of a chore to keep this up. The truth, however, is that there is no standard that we are trying to meet with this; we are not getting graded on this—it is too important to be judged by anyone, and it is a profound business just between us and God. Progress, though perhaps unseen by us at first, is immediate inside of us and we *will* see it after just a short period of practice—the fruits of it will be both *transforming* and "quietly" miraculous. This private exercise, or "struggle," of practicing the presence of God is more than worth it for us. *We* are more than worth it. It is a fast and simple recipe for right living. That's why we keep going, no matter how imperfectly we think we are doing it...or "not" doing it. So, we don't despair or get frustrated and give in to the temptation to stop. *Every* step benefits us; and with just a little bit of practice and persistence, it will become more automatic. ...Slowly, one step and day at a time. If we fall or fail at this, we just quickly get back up and simply confess our faults and feelings, trusting God's unconditional love and power over everything. It's truly about the (guaranteed) progress, not perfection.

As we struggle (or at least try) to do this according to our imperfect ability, we will see that by God's grace the transformation is *already* happening in the journey! Glory be to God and His ways which are beyond all understanding! Praise be to God our Creator, Who is not about theory, ideas, laws, or achievements—He is real and personally present with us at our most basic human level, and He passionately loves us and meets us exactly where we are; He *never* demands too much of us or is inconsiderate of who we are. Jesus Christ, the son of God through whom we and all things were created, came in the flesh to us and interacts with us on our human level face-to-face. (Yes, through others, as well as *inside* us.) We can only live in God; we can only discover reality and satisfaction in Him. And the most direct way is through His son, His "incarnate Love" for us in human form, whom He gave for this purpose. Because...His son Jesus *willingly* died for us, personally, to show us in a very real and historically-rooted "factual" way that God loves each one of us *that* much, as if you or I were the only person in the world for Him. So there is no longer any obstacle (real or imagined in our minds) between God and us, to keep us away from Him. (John 3:16) But what if I am not a Christian or I don't believe in this? Don't let this stop you: We simply ask God (whatever our image and belief of Him may be) to help us understand His love for us more perfectly...and we keep going. We surrender our own ideas, our conclusions, and our "sense" of logic (our arguments), and we invite him in and practice His holy presence with us...in spite of how it feels at first. Faith and understanding and the peace of His mysterious—but most simple and pure—love for us will quickly become more and more clear. So we just keep going. That takes faith and humility, and we ask God for this always because it is our elusive key.

We already have all we need to "acquire" this attitude, because we were created that way. We ask for God's help and start practicing His real presence with us... By a constant and candid conversation with Him and a willingness to look inside ourselves with Him. That means we become willing and trusting to wake up into reality and see that *we* are not God, but that God has something infinitely better for us than we could ever imagine for ourselves. We become like little children, setting aside our "desperate" faith in our own understanding, conclusions, and conditions and by trusting Him; and we start loving one another as we would like God to love us. If we find this difficult at first, we don't worry but just ask for His help. (He is *eagerly* waiting for us to ask Him.) We can then accept His—and *our*—reality. We soon understand with conviction that we exist *in* Him, and nothing is impossible for Him. We become transformed more like the wind: We no longer feel stuck in our problems and bound and shackled by this world and its difficulties. We are truly reborn! (John 3:7-8) We live in the grace of the new covenant and way of life as actual children of God. The answer, practicing the presence of God, is in its simplest form Love—Jesus asks this of us as his only commandment. We are being transformed into creatures of truth; we are waking up into amazing *reality*, and we are ***free!***

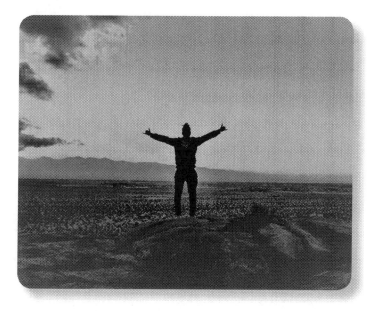

Printed in the United States
By Bookmasters